Reiki Healing:

The Ultimate Step-by-Step, Comprehensive Guide to Master Reiki & Healing Meditation

Copyright © 2019 by Crystal Marcus

All rights reserved. No part of this publication may be reproduced, stored in a retrieval system or transmitted, in **any** form or by **any** means, electronic, mechanical, photocopying, recording or otherwise, without permission in writing from the publisher.

Table of Contents

Reiki Healing: 1
Introduction..5
Chapter 1: Reiki..9

    History of Reiki 12
    The Five Principles of Reiki 20
    The Three Pillars of Reiki 28
    Branches of Reiki.. 41
    Reiki Healing Stories 45

Chapter 2: Reiki Energy 49

    What is Reiki Energy? 49
    How Does the Body Use Reiki Energy?............55
    How Your Life Can Be Improved with Reiki Healing.. 57
    The Energy Meridians of the Human Body.....64
    Reiki and the 7 Chakras 68

Chapter 3: Reiki Symbols....................................94

    About the Reiki Symbols 97
    The Original Reiki Symbols and Meanings......98
    Crystal Work with Reiki.................................112

Chapter 4: Reiki Healing 120

What is the Difference Between Reiki and Other Energy Healing? 120
Preparing Yourself 124
Reiki for Food 131
Healing Ourselves and Others with Reiki 138
Healing Animals with Reiki 145
Reiki Exercises for Beginners 148

Chapter 5: A Little Something More 154

Holy Fire and Other Reiki Branches 154
Reiki and Kundalini Meditation 156

Conclusion 168

Introduction

Congratulations on purchasing *Reiki Healing* and thank you for doing so.

Reiki healing is the concept of using the life force energy within you, focused in such a way that it optimizes the healing benefits that you can apply to yourself, others, animals, the food we eat, and can even be done from a distance!

Reiki is more than just a tool to be used for healing. It can also be used to center, calm, and relax both body and mind. It can be used to revitalize and energize. It can strengthen your body, such as your lungs and circulation through the proper use of breathing techniques and meditation. It helps you to become more aware, and increases your concentration levels.

Through the hand and finger techniques, combined with the use Reiki symbol practice, it increases your finer motor skills, coordination, and reflexes.

On the actual healing side of things, the possibilities and benefits are endless. Besides general healing, it can also help to relieve pain and reduce discomfort. You can use it to purify toxins from your body, or that of others. The stress reduction benefits alone help to contribute to a better health overall!

This book is here to help you get started with the understanding of Reiki, how it works, how you can use it, and actually get you on your way to healing with Reiki energy. Any kind of energy healing takes time. Daily practice makes your energy connection and use stronger and more effective.

There are many ways that energy healing can be practiced, and working with Reiki energy is no exception. There is no one, true way. Working with energy, especially healing energy, is a personal experience. You will get the most out of it, and achieve the greatest results when you are familiar and comfortable with what you are doing and how you are doing it.

Relax, take your time. Try practicing at the same time every day, or work at different times of the day until you find the time that suits you best. Dress comfortably. Work with it when you know you won't be disturbed.

Don't force it, allow the energy and how you work with it to come naturally. You don't have to make or create a ritual surrounding your energy work and/or preparation, but working regularly does help increase your abilities at a faster rate.

While there is no true right or wrong way to work with Reiki energy, when done correctly, it does produce better results. When you feel ready to take the next step, find a class under a Reiki Master, or a local practitioner who may be willing to help show you some of the best ways to manage the techniques you are learning.

Reiki doesn't just work for physical healing, although that is often what draws the initial practitioner. Reiki energy can be used for emotional healing, mental healing, and spiritual healing. As with any energy work, the more you put into it, the more you will get out of it. The better care you take of yourself and your body, the better the energy will flow through you, and the better clarity you will find to direct it towards whatever it is you choose to use it for. Eating healthy, developing regular exercise, even if it is just simple stretching, getting a good night's sleep… these are all things that can help you prepare your body and keep it clear for the Reiki energy to flow through you better as a conduit.

Take the time to go through the book in its entirety, so that you gain a good comprehension of the journey upon which you are choosing to embark. Then go back through and study it further in depth, and start working with some of the tips, techniques, and exercises to get you going on your way to practice working with Reiki energy.

There are plenty of books on this subject on the market, thanks again for choosing this one! Every effort was made to ensure it is full of as much useful information as possible, please enjoy!

Chapter 1: Reiki

Modern day Reiki is alternative medicine style of healing, using Universal Life Force energy. It is the use of Universal Life energy, channeled through the practitioner and out the hands, or palms, to perform emotional, spiritual, or physical healing on the subject/client. In Japanese, "Rei" translates to "life force" or "universe", indicating an outside source. "Ki", also referred to as "chi" or "qi", describes the life force energy of the physical body. So together, "Rei-ki" is universal life force energy.

Reiki is a form of metaphysical healing, and while it utilizes the Universal Life Force, or qi (or chi), there has been no "scientific" proof of the existence of this life force energy. However, scientific proof or not, under the name, qi, it has been used for thousands of years by both Chinese and Japanese practitioners, and as general life force energy, for possibly even more. That it is still in continued use to this day, speaks volumes for the validity of this use of energy for healing.

This is not a religious or spiritual form of healing, nor is it any form of massage or other therapeutic touch, or hypnosis, and neither is it based on the premise of suggestion. It does not matter what your belief system is, how intelligent you are, or even whether you actually believe in the concept for it to work.

Reiki is available for everyone to learn. It doesn't depend on your level of spiritual development. That being said, you are open as a channel for the Universal Life Force energy when you are open and working in a way that is harmonious and balanced with others.

The purpose of Reiki is to help the body work its own healing through the use of energy. The practitioner is actually giving the body the energy it needs to help work its own healing. Sometimes this can be a more generalized energy, sometimes a more directed energy, depending on what the intent of the practitioner is, and what the body will take from it and actually use.

All things contain a life force energy. It flows freely through our bodies, and that of all living things, even plants and animals. When we are at optimum health, the energy flows freely through our bodies, and we are charged and ready to go. When it gets blocked or weakens, it weakens our overall health and energy levels, allowing for ailments of all kinds, mental, emotional, spiritual, and physical to occur, because our energy isn't strong enough to fight them off, or prevent them from happening. It causes our bodies and selves, to become out of balance.

When our life force energy is at lower levels, we are more apt to feel stress, depression, and occur illnesses. When our life force energy is at higher levels, our capability for feeling healthy and happy increases.

Most of us, in this modern world, continually run on empty, trying to accomplish everything we need to do within short periods of time. We constantly deplete our life force energies. It stresses us out, and doesn't allow for any energy left to keep our bodies in a healthier state. Thus, the Reiki practitioner provides the extra life force energy needed to stay at higher levels, aiding in stress reduction and relaxation, which puts our bodies in a better state for healing at deeper levels.

Some practitioners actually touch their subjects, while others do not. Because of this, make sure to check the laws in your location regarding Reiki, as some states have passed laws that require a massage license to perform Reiki in a practitioner setting, even though you are not actually touching or performing massage on your client.

History of Reiki

The history of Reiki contains much more importance than just a general passing knowledge of how Reiki came into being. Reiki has been passed down through generations of teachers. Each student of Reiki, when properly attuned by a Master, is added to the lineage of the Reiki line. Every traditional Reiki Master can actually state their place in the lineage of Reiki, based on their teacher, and their teacher's teacher, and that lineage can be traced back to the original progenitor of Reiki, Mikao Usui.

Mikao Usui was born in a small village to a once influential and well-known samurai family in Japan on August 15, 1865. Because he was a descendant of an old samurai family, he was able to receive a more privileged education than he would have otherwise, coming from such humble beginnings. He was raised on Buddhist teachings by his family, and gained his initial education from a Tendai Monastery.

His martial arts training began when he was 12, where he gained high ranks and levels of proficiency. He spoke multiple languages and became highly knowledgeable in philosophy, theology, and in the field of medicine. Mikao Usui also learned *Kiko*, which is the Japanese form of *Chi Kung*, which is a Chinese form of cultivating life force energy, as well as samurai swordsmanship. He went on to become a Buddhist teacher, and had the respect of both peers and students.

Usui's true passion and interest lay in finding a way to heal others, as well as himself. His goal was to find a way to use life force energy without depleting it, and being able to do so through a method using his hands for channeling the energy. He spent many years devoted to this task of discovering a new system that could benefit humanity. He took a very open-minded approach, searching within all modalities and religions, which is why Reiki has no religious attachment, and is open and available to all for use.

His search and studies took him into all modalities, including that of Western medicine. Eventually, he returned to his original Buddhist teachings, still seeking his answer. He returned to the original Tendai temple of his youth, and became a Buddhist Monk.

It was during his time spent at the Tendai temple that he undertook a special 21-day instructional course on seeking enlightenment, *Isyu Guo*. It involved visiting Mount Kurama and staying in a cave there, praying, meditating and fasting for those days. Nothing happened until the final, 21st day, when he received a vision that involving ancient Sanskrit symbols. His moment of enlightenment had come. With this vision, he saw a way that these symbols could be incorporated and used to develop the healing system he had been seeking for all those years.

It is said, even on his memorial stone in Japan, that when this enlightenment occurred, that a great source of energy appeared over his head and infused him with an unlimited supply of life force energy, and the ability to impart this energy to others. It was what could be considered the very first, Divine Reiki attunement.

After the vision on Mount Kurama, Usui returned to civilization in Kyoto and set up a clinic where he began to use his new technique to heal people, while also teaching others the modality, so that they, too, could use this new and amazing technique. It became so successful, that he was able to travel across Japan to teach his Reiki methodology. He offered inexpensive healing, sometimes even for free, so that everyone could benefit from his healing techniques.

He also taught Reiki to others, helping them learn how to heal themselves and replenish their life force energies. His primary focus was that of teaching others how to heal themselves, before all else. He built this premise with the sound belief that you first have to be able to heal yourself and be whole, before you can work to heal others.

Mikao Usui died March 9, 1926, but not before training over 20 Reiki Masters in his modality, the symbols, and the method of attunement so that his legacy of healing would live on. One of these Reiki Masters was Dr. Chujiro Hayashi.

Chujiro Hayashi was born in 1879. He was once an officer in the Imperial Navy, and a surgeon trained in both Chinese and Western Medicines. He met Mikao Usui in 1925, and studied with him for 10 months before Usui's death in 1926, receiving his teacher's training in Reiki, and becoming one of the Reiki Masters of Usui's lineage. After the death of

Usui, it is said that Hayashi became the leader of Reiki.

While working with the Reiki modality taught to him by Usui, Hayashi started to develop a more methodical approach with science-based techniques, and introduced hand positions and attunement to the original modality, with Usui's permission. Chujiro Hayashi published a guide to his new and combined teachings, the Hayashi Healing Guide.

Hayashi opened a small clinic for Reiki healing and teaching near the Imperial Palace in Toyko. When he accepted a student into teaching the modality of Reiki, he had several things that he insisted on as part of the training that he offered. One was that his students work with Reiki daily, and the other was to volunteer hours in the clinic to use the skills they were being taught, a sort of "internship" to the Reiki practice.

When it appeared as though Japan would be entering into World War II, Hayashi took his own life on May 10, 1940. He knew with the entering into the World War, that he, as an officer and surgeon, would be recalled to duty. He could not abide by the thought of taking a life, so he ended his. By the time of his death, Hayashi had trained 14 Reiki Masters. The lineage of most Western Reiki Masters comes from him through one of his students, Mrs. Hawayo Takata.

Mrs. Hawayo Takata was a woman of Japanese descent born in Hawaii in 1900. She was in Tokyo in 1935 when she became very ill after the death of her husband and daughter, and was told she was in need of surgery. Going on her instincts, she asked her doctor whether he knew of any alternative medicine treatments that would work for her condition. She was directed to Dr. Hayashi, at his Reiki practice.

Regardless of her skepticism, she made an appointment, and after her initial consult, she saw Dr. Hayashi daily. She found rest and relaxation, and to her surprise, healing. She went on to study Reiki techniques under Dr. Hayashi from 1936-

1938, and became a Reiki Master under his teachings.

It was Mrs. Takata who was the primary source of the Reiki lineage in the Western part of the world. She brought the teachings back with her to Hawaii. After a visit from Dr. Hayashi to see her Reiki clinic, she was attuned as a Master herself, and Dr. Hayashi passed the leadership torch of Reiki onto her. She made her own changes to the Reiki practice, and began spreading the healing practice even more.

Mrs. Takata continued teaching and healing with Reiki for over 40 years. She began training additional Reiki Masters in the 1970s. At the time of her passing, December 11, 1980, there were an additional 22 Reiki Masters trained by her. These teachers took Reiki and spread its teachings in the West. Without Mrs. Takata, Reiki may have never gained the recognition in the United States that it has, and we would have not benefitted from its miraculous healing energies.

It is important to note that Reiki has adapted and evolved through the use of each student to Master. It is a system that is not static, although it can be, but rather, it adapts and flows, much like the energy used. It is well suited for healing many in this way, but most of all, starting with the self. This is one of the prerequisites of becoming a Reiki practitioner, and eventually a Reiki Master... the use of Reiki to heal and balance yourself, so that you are much better suited, and a far better channel for the healing of others.

On the grounds of the Saihoji Temple in Tokyo, a memorial stone ten feet high and four feet wide was erected in 1927, dedicated to the life of Mikao Usui. His life is beautifully written in Kanji, a fitting tribute to a man who brought so much healing to the world. Written on the stone are also teachings, in particular, the "5 Admonitions", which have come to be known as the 5 Principles of Reiki.

The Five Principles of Reiki

Hatsurei-Ho is a Japanese meditation practice that incorporates meditation on the five principles of

Reiki. Usui developed the five principles of Reiki, originally known as the 5 Admonitions. These principles were developed by Mikao Usui as a way to bring balance and harmony to your life every day.

The five principles are recommended to be focused on each day, but strict adherence is not necessary. There should be no guilt for not practicing or focusing on the five principles. In fact, part of the principles and the idea behind them is to release guilt, anger, sorrow, and stress from your life to better open yourself as a channel for the healing Reiki energy to flow through and replenish your system, so that you in turn can better heal others.

So, let's take a look at the five principles of Reiki, as taught by Mikao Usui and written on his memorial stone. These are rough translations, based on the original Kanji, and personified by Western ways of thinking and thought.

It begins with...

Kyo dake wa... Just for today.

The practice of the five principles takes life one day at a time, with no focus on the past or future. This gets into the practice of the five principles by taking each principle one day at a time, just for the day that you are currently living. Just for today…

Okolu-na… Don't get angry.

Another way to think of this is… I will release all of my anger, and angry thoughts. Just for today, I will not be angry.

In order for energy flow to not be hindered, we need the ability to maintain control of our emotions. We need to gain an understanding of what triggers our emotions, in this case, anger. Anger or having angry thoughts about someone or something gives it control over us. When we are not in control, our energy becomes sluggish or blocked. It does not move properly through us.

By learning to turn anger into a positive thing, or by responding in a positive manner, we retain control, and our energy or power is not given to another, or to anything else. In every situation, with every person, we need to approach it with compassion.

There is usually something that lies beneath the surface that gives cause to fuel our anger. By discovering what it is that is triggering our anger beneath the surface, we can aptly avoid such a feeling or focus of our energy in the future. By recognizing it for what it is, we learn to stop it before it starts, and gives us a new way of understanding.

Our new way of looking at how we perceive things helps us to not dwell on the negative aspects of life and allows us to surround ourselves with positive things, positive moments, and positive people.

Shinpai Suna... Don't be grievous.

This is one of those phrases where translation can be difficult between Eastern and Western philosophies and ways of thought. The Western way of thinking has interpreted this as... Do not worry.

Another way of looking at it is... I release all thoughts of worry and fear. Just for today, I will not worry.

An imbalance of the emotions, mind, body, and spirit can occur when we worry. It brings levels of anxiety, fear, and stress into our lives that work against the free-flowing energy necessary for healing ourselves and others.

Instead of allowing ourselves to worry, we need to turn our focus to viewing obstacles and fears into opportunities for growth and learning. In this way, we approach life with a positive attitude, and leave our worries behind, letting them go.

Kansha shite... Express your gratitude.

Another way to look at this is... Give thanks for the many blessings you have in your life. I will be thankful for the many things that I have in my life. Just for today... I am grateful.

All too often our focus is on what we don't have in our lives, what is missing. When we actually take a moment to pause, or stop, and contemplate what we *do* have in our lives, the picture usually looks far more positive.

This is not just about those material things, the things that money buys us. It is time to take stock of what we do have in our lives… family, health, friends, freedom, knowledge, wisdom… the list can go on. When you stop to contemplate these things, you will be amazed at the number of things you may find that you actually have in your life for which to be grateful.

Goo hage me… Be diligent in your business.

This is another hard to interpret based on Eastern-Western differences in ways of thinking. In Western thought, it has basically been interpreted as… Work hard and work honestly. Some forms of Reiki teachings have totally changed this particular principle to modernize it in the form of… I expand my consciousness.

As noted in the history section of Reiki, the face of Reiki is constantly changing and evolving. This form of the principle may not be written on the memorial stone, but it hard to contemplate that Mikao Usui would have found any fault with the premise.

Be diligent in your business... Always approach your work to the best of your abilities. Be open to the flow and to sharing the benefit of your talents and gifts with all those around you. When you hold back, you cheat others, but you also cheat yourself of the gift of giving, or the truth that you are possessed of these amazing gifts and talents at all.

Hito ni shinsetsu ni... Be kind to others.

In any language or way of thought, this is similar, and is something we should strive to practice, Reiki or not. By giving goodness and kindness, we receive goodness and kindness in return. This is the principle of Karmic law. Or, more aptly, it is the principle of Dharmic law.

When our thoughts are positive, we bring positive things into our lives. At the very least, more things that we can feel positive about come into our lives. It is our choice on how to view them. But the transverse is also true. Negativity and negative thoughts will bring those same things into our lives.

It is not only the concept of Mikao Usui and his Reiki teachings. By reflecting on these principles daily, or even at all regularly, and putting them to work in your life, you will bring positive change into your world. When done in concert with the teachings of Reiki, the benefit is even greater.

With or without Reiki, these principles are something that we should all strive to live by. In truth, it is the first step of Reiki, at the very beginning—learning to heal yourself and affect positive change in your life. Reiki is a way of life and healing that has touched thousands of people. Usui students, at all their various levels of attunement, numbered over 2,000. Hayashi and Takata have expended that even further. Even without Reiki, these five principles will not only help you to improve your life, but it will help to improve the lives of all those around you with whom you come into contact.

The Three Pillars of Reiki

The three pillars of Reiki are different than the five principles. The five principles set us up for gaining better energy, better healing, and better overall quality of life for ourselves and those we touch, with or without the Reiki energy coming into play or focus.

Mindfulness in meditation, a focus on what you are doing with the energy, connecting to the energy, what you are about to do with the energy… that is a big part of the practice of Reiki. With mindfulness, it creates a better flow for the healing energy, and it brings more meaning to the Reiki session.

The three pillars are necessary to the practice and implementation of Reiki. These three, as taught by Mikao Usui, are *Gassho*, *Reiji-Ho*, and *Chiryo*. These are foundational practices developed by Usui to bring the best use of the Reiki energy during the healing session. Each has multiple purposes, which include...

- Cleansing the energy, a sort of "spiritual hygiene" to bring a centered state of calm to the practitioner's mind before implementing a Reiki session.

- To assist in letting go of the practitioner's ego. This allows for the practitioner to not put their thoughts on what needs to be done into the session, but rather, allows for them to be open and receptive to receiving intuitive information from the source of the Reiki energy itself, or to Divine Guidance, opening themselves as a channel to the energy, rather than directing the energy to where they "think" it should go.

- To connect the practitioner to the Reiki energy for healing.

- It helps the practitioner to work from a more intuitive place when sending the Reiki energy in a direction that best benefits the healing process.

- It helps to create a "sacred space" for the Reiki session that puts the practitioner in a place of mindfulness and focus that benefits the healing process.

The First Pillar: *Gassho*

Gassho is the first pillar of Reiki. It is a meditative practice, and yet more. It is *Gassho* that cleanses the energy of the practitioner, and sets focus and the intention for the Reiki healing session. It helps the practitioner to set aside their ego, and it initiates an invitation to the Reiki energy to come in and ignite the healing energy for the session that is about to take place.

In Westernized Reiki, *Gassho* is taught as a seemingly simple meditation practice that involves the Reiki practitioner holding their hands in a sort of prayer position and then spending their focus on the point where the middle fingertips meet. While this is in part the process, it is actually more involved than that. The fingertips only act as a focal point in the physical, to help keep the practitioner in a moment of mindfulness. As the skill level develops, the Reiki practitioner is able to take the mindfulness they find with *Gassho* and combine it with their intention, as well as breath work to help strengthen the Reiki energies for their use.

For Cleansing. The best use of *Gassho* for cleansing is to spend 5 to 10 minutes putting themselves in a state of mindfulness to be open to the positive aspects and guidance of the Reiki energy. This is something that should be done before every session, and in-between sessions. It is a time to let the rest of their life focus slip away, and devote themselves to the task of energy work at hand. This is also the time where the Reiki practitioner can clear any blockages or sluggishness to their energy and energy channels, and cleanse the space around them for the healing that needs to take place.

Take the time to focus on the space around you and perform any "rituals" you normally do before any kind of spiritual or energy work. This can be using Reiki symbols for clearing, smudging the space, or the burning of other herbs or incense, sending pink, loving light, or cleansing white light… whatever you are most connected to, as that is where your energies of purification are going to be at their strongest.

Find a comfortable sitting position and start your breathing techniques to calm your mind. As you calm yourself, bring your focus to the point where your middle fingertips of your hand meet when holding them in a prayer position in front of you.

Feel the space around you filling with the Reiki energy, calling it in to fill you and all of the space around you. Let it flow into your body with your breath, filling your entire being. As you're breathing, exhale any stress or negativity that you may feel. It doesn't belong with you, and it doesn't belong in the session of healing you are about to enter.

Take as much time as you need, whether it be five minutes, ten, or longer. We are human. Some days it may take us longer than others to properly put ourselves in the place needed to channel the Reiki energy and be open to Divine Guidance for its use. Make sure that you let go of your ego. Until it is gone, a proper healing cannot take place. Keep at it until you feel completely centered, calm and at peace. It is only when you can find this place of balance and centeredness that you should invite the individual in need of the healing into the space you have created for them and for yourself to work with them.

Setting Intention, Inviting & Igniting the Reiki Energy. When the individual to be healed has entered your cleansed and prepared space, take the time to consult with them now that your ego has stepped aside. When you feel that they have indicated all that they can, have them lay comfortably in the place you have prepared, whether it be a table, couch, the floor... whatever space that you work within. Come to the head of the person you are healing, and enter your state of *Gassho* mindfulness again. This time, allow your focus to be on whatever it was that you and the individual to be healed discussed, and bring the energies in for the greatest and highest good of the individual. Feel again the Reiki energy gathering around you and breathe it in, allowing it to feel you completely on all levels of your being. When you feel completely connected and filed with the Reiki energy, invite it to come into your hands to work with the healing energy. When you can feel its presence igniting the healing energy within your hands, it is time to begin.

Returning to Mindfulness, or Need of Further Guidance. During the Reiki healing session, you can return to your state of *Gassho* mindfulness at any time. It is a place of safety where you can reset your focus, intention, or allow yourself to be open for guidance from the Reiki energy as to what to do and where to place your hands for the healing session.

Gassho is the place which anchors you during a Reiki healing session, which is primarily intuitive. Sometimes you need to ground to understand where you are at with the healing process. If you feel an energy shift, or your mind or consciousness starts to feel as though its going astray from the task at hand, re-enter the space of *Gassho* and find your center.

Return to the head of the individual to re-center your energies and focus. Ask the Reiki energy for guidance in what you are doing. Watch for signs that may be guiding you... a thought that comes to mind, feeling drawn to a certain area, a shift of energy, part of the body lighting up in your subconscious Third Eye... Pay attention to the guidance being offered. Just flow with the energy as it flows through you. Allow it to guide you in what you need to do.

Gassho is a safe space that can be returned to any time during a session if you feel uncertain as to what to do next, or just need to re-center and refocus.

Giving Thanks and Returning from the Energy. At the close of a Reiki healing session, you may find yourself wanting to return to *Gassho* again. If so, instead of placing yourself at the head of the individual, move to place yourself at their feet. Allow yourself to give thanks to the Reiki energy for its presence. Thank both it and the individual that you have been healing for allowing you to be the channel for the energy to bring the greatest and highest good into being. Ask for the energy to release from the individual, from the space, and from you. See the connection gently releasing and the energy leaving. When you feel that this has been accomplished, ground yourself to bring yourself back into the space of the world around you.

The Second Pillar: *Reiji-Ho*

Reiji-Ho is the second pillar of Reiki. *Gassho* is the primary pillar of Reiki, and you will see parts and elements of *Gassho* throughout the other two pillars. *Reiji-Ho* is the pillar that focuses primarily on asking for guidance from the Reiki and Universal energies. Working with the hand positions can be very important for those who are first learning Reiki, as they give something to bring your focus to in order to keep you in a mindful state of being as you work with the Reiki energy.

As a practitioner becomes more practiced and comfortable with their state of mindfulness, they can then begin to work more intuitively, which is what working with Reiki energy is truly about. When uncertain of how to work intuitively, returning to work with the Reiki hand positions can be a good way to fall back and reset your focus and intention.

When working with *Reiji-Ho*, you are inviting guidance in to help you do the greatest and highest good with the energy work you are doing. The *Reiji-Ho* starts with the *Gassho* position, hands held in the prayer position, while asking of the Universe and Reiki energies to guide your hands and use of energy to the greatest and highest good of the individual for which you are performing the healing. You then wait, in a place of mindfulness, listening with all of your senses for an answer to your supplication.

Pay attention for any and all responses. Watch for any response from the individual for which you are doing the healing. Listen to the thoughts that pass through your mind, see what your eyes perceive, even the spiritual sight from your Third Eye. Feel any responses that your own body may have.

Let go of your ego and empty your mind of conscious thoughts that you may have directing you toward action. Allow yourself to become an open vessel for the guidance and energy to flow through to effect the best and highest healing possible during the session. It can take time, but as you practice *Reji-Ho*, you will learn how you work with the energy and guidance, in what forms it takes to show you the way. It is an intuitive process, and we all perceive things differently from one another. There is no right or wrong way to receive or perceive how you are being guided.

Trust in yourself, in the Divine Guidance being sent to you, and in the individual, you are working to heal is needed when using *Reiji-Ho*. Mindfulness is a necessity! It requires a lot of trust to open yourself and allow yourself to become a vessel, or channel, for the energy to come through, without ego stepping in the way to direct it.

You must trust in your perception of what is being sent to you for guidance, and act accordingly as you receive it, to work toward the greatest and highest good. Know that what you are doing is being done as it is needed. If you feel yourself coming out of the space of *Reji-Ho* and losing your place and space of being a guided vessel or channel for the healing energy, reset yourself with *Gassho* and move back into the space of *Reji-Ho*.

The Third Pillar: *Chiryo*

Chiryo is the third pillar of Reiki. *Chiryo* is all about the action of the Reiki energy. From Japanese, *Chiryo* is translated into "treatment", and is the primary focus of every Reiki healing treatment session. When first learning Reiki, many new practitioners focus on the position of their hand placements, and just open themselves, trusting that the Reiki energy will do what it needs to. And in some small part, it will.

As confidence and comfort levels grow, and the practitioner deepens their understanding and become more involved in their practice of using Reiki energy, they discover the connection between *Reji-Ho*, the guidance they receive, and how that guidance can change the direction of the energy flow, dependent upon the greatest and highest good, and need, of the individual being healed.

When truly connected to the third pillar of *Chiryo*, the practitioner will often move past the use of the initial hand positions they are taught, and sometimes even past the use of hands.

It is because of this that Reiki has changed and developed through different practitioner, even to include the earliest Masters, Hayashi and Takata. Usui knew this. It is why he did not stop the teachings of his initial modality developed to change and evolve. We must all allow ourselves the fluidity to be like the energy and flow where needed and guided.

Branches of Reiki

It is unclear as to how many different branches they truly are when it comes to the teachings of Reiki. The originations of Reiki came from Mikao Usui, and have been passed down through the lineages of his students. Once the teachings of Reiki came to Western civilization, they sometimes took on different meanings, as the translation in the New Age of energy work didn't always translate to the lineage teachings of the original Master.

Reiki began as a modality developed and defined, in specifics. As time has passed, the modality has come to incorporate different energy work that does not have the same basis as the original teachings of Usui. This is not to say that any of these "branches" are any less valid in their success rates of healing and providing the highest and greatest good for those in need of healing.

But because Reiki was allowed by its originator to "evolve" and change as Divine inspiration came through each Master, there are times where this evolution has actually degenerated the true, initial form of Usui's teachings, rather than enhancing what was already developed. It is the difference between receiving Divine Inspiration from the source of energy, the Universal Life Force, or allowing ego to step in and direct how the modality should be changed.

A Reiki branch, in essence, is developed any time a change is made to the way the Reiki energy is used by a Master, and passed down through their teachings to their subsequent students. Because of the development of so many different branches of Reiki, it is easier to put them into categories for classification, rather than to list the thousands of different branches that are out there. Even the Reiki Source Guide lists a minimum of several dozen.

Reiki Classifications

Japanese Reiki: Although the original definition of Japanese Reiki was set as taught in Japan by someone born in Japan, dedicated to the purity of the original Mikao Usui modality, this has been expanded to include the teaching of the original Japanese style of Reiki, even if taught by someone of Western origins.

Western Reiki: These branches of Reiki usually come through the lineage of Mrs. Hawayo Takata, and teach her branch of Usui-style Reiki, usually taught by someone of Western origins, but also taught by some of the more contemporary Japanese.

Tibetan Reiki: This is the teaching of traditional Usui-style Reiki that has evolved, or changed, through the addition of new Tibetan symbols and other elements.

Eastern Reiki: Eastern Reiki is that which has been evolved and changed based on beliefs of a more contemporary India-style of teachings, enhanced with Chakra work, aura healing, and sometimes even involving some Hindu deities.

Seichem Reiki: Seichem Reiki treats the Reiki energy as the elemental energy of earth, and incorporates the other elements (Seichim) of air, fire, water, as well as incorporating other concepts that flow with that energy system.

Non-Traditional Reiki: These sometimes have dubious origins. While some adhere at least in part to the teachings of Mikao Usui, others incorporate what they consider to be the Reiki energy as something different, in more of a New Age fashion of use, which can include the use of crystals, dragons, angels, supernatural beings, elements, etc. While not necessarily fraudulent in their application and/or success, they have strayed far enough from Usui's teachings to be considered pure forms of Reiki as far as the traditionalists are concerned. They tend more toward using the name Reiki to describe the energy as a spiritual energy used for healing, rather than a Universal energy separate from spirituality or religion. But as we said from the beginning, there is no right or wrong way to practice Reiki.

Reiki Healing Stories

There are many healing stories that come as a testament to the power of Reiki. Several are listed here just to demonstrate the miraculous healing energy power of Reiki, even on those not present!

Delores
Delores had experienced chronic pain for years. It was so excruciating that she could barely stand to get out of bed each day. She decided one day to go to an event to learn about what Reiki healing was all about.

She sat through part of the event, and her pain started to reach an unbearable point. It got so bad at one point, that she almost left. Something made her stay. At the end of the lecture part of the teaching of what Reiki was all about, the speaker invited those in the room to come up for a brief Reiki treatment, to experience the energy for themselves.

Skeptical, but figuring there was nothing to be lost, Delores waited her turn, and then went to receive her 5-minute Reiki treatment. She was amazed. Almost instantly, she felt relief from the pain, something that she had definitely not expected! As the day went on, she felt more and more like her joints had been renewed, and her muscles loosened, something that had never happened before, even with deep massage. The next morning, Delores did not have to struggle getting out of bed, and actually found enjoyment for her day. She now receives regular Reiki treatments, and feels as though she has gained a new lease and love for life.

Manuel

Yvonne was working one day at a department store. A gentleman in a nearby aisle started to look very pale and shaky. A Reiki practitioner, Yvonne went over to inquire whether he was all right. Manuel nodded, and indicated that he was experiencing all too common signs that indicated he had a seizure coming on.

At a loss, because Manuel begged her not to call an ambulance because his insurance wouldn't cover it, she took Manuel to a waiting area outside the dressing rooms where he could sit. Not knowing what else to do, she placed her hands on his back and started channeling Reiki energy for a brief treatment.

Manuel stopped shaking and his body went from rigid to relaxed. He told Yvonne that he had never had a seizure stop once it had progressed that far before, and usually felt sick afterwards. Not only had Yvonne's use of Reiki energy stopped the seizure in its tracks, but it also prevented Manuel from becoming ill, as was normal for him. He was very grateful for Yvonne's energy work with Reiki that day!

Matt
Amanda's boyfriend, Matt, had her over for dinner one evening. As he was pulling dinner out of the oven, the pan began to tip, and without thinking, he grabbed it with his unprotected other hand. His

hand was burned on his pam and two out of his four fingers, as well as his thumb.

Even after running it under cold water, by the end of dinner, those spots were bright red and started to blister. Amanda decided to perform some Reiki on it for him, and although not expecting any results, he did admit to her that it seemed to take the edge off the pain.

The next morning, Amanda called in to check on Matt, and totally amazed and blown away, he admitted that he not only had no pain, but there was also no redness nor signs of blisters!

Chapter 2: Reiki Energy

Now that we have covered the concepts of Reiki and its history, we now turn to a deeper look at what Reiki is and how we can use it for our own benefit, and for the benefit of others.

What is Reiki Energy?

It is probably best if we start with energy and what that is. Energy itself is defined in many different ways by many different disciplines. Everything from spiritual and religious practices, all the way to the scientific properties of physics, energy seems to be everywhere.

Energy equals mass squared times the speed of light. That is Einstein defining the universe with physics. Starting by defining energy of course. We can define energy and energies in a spiritual way as well. The breath of god, or the life of a plant, can all be traced back to basic energies.

Energy defined leans to strength and vitality. This is the stuff of work to sustain activity. Vigor and liveliness lead to this vitality. It is the fire and passion of what makes us do what we do.

When dealing with perspective and different ways of thought, it is reasonable to say that Eastern society looks at the spirit of life differently than the West, we have to take into account that Reiki comes from this Eastern way of thinking.

It may seem strange at first to look at the Eastern philosophy as this his blend of color and life and energy resides in all things. The Universe resides in all things. Energy is the Universe. The Universe is energy. Back and forth the energies flow.

If you have ever sat in a field of flowers and grass, with the sun making you all warm, you begin to feel this energy. It is the buzzing and sound of the insects around you. It is the flittering of a small butterfly as it floats by.

The energies of us as we live is also a way of measuring this energy. Imagine your life as a shell with no energy. Our lives are powered up by our own energies. Without energy we are just a husk. Yes, there is something to be said for not believing. It is only in the moments that we see ourselves for what we are with and without.

Energy is.

With this in mind we can begin to extrapolate as to what the energies of life are. Once we leave the debate of the mystical spiritual conflict versus cold, demanding, clinical science behind, we can begin to see life for what it is. A series of energy movements.

This philosophy is a corner stone in describing what Reiki energy is and what it does.

Consider the fact that energy can be either flowing or not, then we can begin to see that those who have a skill set can manipulate this energy. This manipulation is not a negative practice. Reiki tends to teach flow over stagnation, or non-flow.

This is what the Reiki energies are. Just as there are so many different life energies, there are so many ways to control your own, as well as that of others.

There is a pattern to life, and to the energies of all forms. Rei, in its spirit and energies, lead us into a pattern of wisdom. This symbol of Rei is an intelligence. A non-physical energy that leads us to a pattern of life. It is an instructor as well as inspiration. It is the higher knowing of what happens and why it happens.

The beginning of Reiki is the why life happens the way it does. This is the energy pattern of why life happens the way it does. Rei is our starting point. Energy and passion combined with intelligence giving us the result of wisdom.

Reiki energy, literally starts with wisdom.

And now the power part. Ki. With the understanding of Ki, we begin to see spirit as power. Ever met someone who is so full of spirit and they seem like they are lit up like a lightbulb? It is when we stop to look around us, that we begin to see that every one of us, every*thing* around us, has this power.

This spirit of Ki is connected to almost everything. Consider the lifeless form of your cellphone. It is just plastic, glass, battery and circuits. There is really no life there. Even when we power it up with energy there is still a lifeless quality to it.

It is when we breathe our Ki into our devices that they become something so much more than a box of plastic. They interact with us in return. Energy is exchanged back and forth. This is the power of the Ki in a more physical form.

We are attached to almost everything. Some expert theologians say we are connected to everything. There is the possibility that Ki does indeed connect us to it all.

This power comes with examination. Once we find the energy of Reiki, we can see if we are flowing with it or not. It is more than acceptable to remain in a state of non-flow with Ki energy and live a full life.

The energy of Reiki is a bit more than just getting by. The energy is about connection and ability to self-heal, and to ultimately heal others. It is about the universe and that flower growing in that pot over there. It is about why our hands move and why we are the way we do.

Ki is power. Power is energy. Life is energy. Life is Ki, for the lack of a better way of defining it.

The energy of Reiki is this pattern that comes from wisdom and can be manipulated within others. Imagine an entire society that is constantly flowing with this energy. What would it accomplish? How would everyone get along?

There is a way to constantly sustain this energy flow. This is the technique of the Reiki, to get us to flow energy. We are not here to remove tumors or cure cancer, although within the realm of Reiki healing, this is possible. We are here to use this energy to get the person who is need of healing to flow with their life force again; to get ourselves flowing again.

This is totally possible. Energy is real. Reiki energy is real. The world around us flows with energy, and we only need to learn how to tap into it, connect, listen, and find our way to move with the flow of the energy for the highest and greatest good of ourselves and others.

How Does the Body Use Reiki Energy?

The use of Reiki energy is intuitive. Our body is comprised of natural energy lines that flow within, invisible to the naked eye, but known by healing practitioners for centuries, long before Reiki even came into being as a healing modality. We call on the Reiki energy to heal ourselves, or to heal others, but we do not direct the energy, we allow it to flow naturally to where it needs to go for the highest and greatest healing of the one who is in need of healing.

The energy flows from the Universal Life force, the source of Reiki energy, into the practitioner when called upon for use. The practitioner, without ego involved, or in the way, allows themselves to be used as a channel for this healing energy. They may be mindful, they may have an idea in mind of what to do with the energy, and bring that thought into being as part of the channeling process, but ultimately, the practitioner steps out of the way and just allows for the Reiki energy to flow through them to the body in need of healing.

Once directed to the intended target, the Reiki energy works with the natural flow of energies within the body to start the healing process. Often times, merely getting the energy of the individual unstuck from its state of non-flow into a state of freely flowing again is enough to facilitate a healing for the individual. Sometimes it takes more than that.

It is not up to us to decide. The body becomes an open receptacle for the energy to come in, and the Reiki energy then works with the body and its natural flows to facilitate the healing process. To try and force something that isn't meant to be can result in a lack of completion, may have no result at all, or in some very few cases, can even be damaging. The Reiki energy, along with the body, knows what is needed and uses Divine guidance to lead the practitioner to the proper movement and healing that needs to take place.

How Your Life Can Be Improved with Reiki Healing

Healing is not a magic pill that is swallowed and your life goes back to normal. For some this is the dream of modern medicine making us all live forever. Once again, beliefs are up to the individual. In our case and in the current state of affairs a pill is not necessarily healing.

Healing is a process. As defined by the word, healing is a process to get back to health. Each individual knows what health is and is not for their own personal life. It is only when we sit down with ourselves and take a look, or understand how we feel, do we find whether we are healthy or not.

Healthy can be a mental state as well. Or an emotional or spiritual one. The physical is not alone in the world of health. We are learning that curing the body sometimes and often starts with the mind.

With that in mind, consider that mental healthiness is something that can bring us to a place of better health and better life.

We are going to look at both the mental and the physical and how Reiki touches and effects each. This is not saying that modern forms of Western, or allopathic medicine has no place in life. Common sense dictates that if we are to make it to a nice ripe old age, we need to consider what is best for each of us and attune our lives to each situation. Most alternative methods of healing can be better served when done in conjunction with these traditional forms of medicine.

Reiki is energy working. This is not something that can be measured with modern medicine tools. Result can play into science. When an individual receives Reiki and improves health, modern medicine can indeed record this. In fact, it can be labelled as empirical data for study and proof of theory.

Is there a value in healing?

Well, beginning with ourselves, we have to consider that we generally want to become healthier overall. Life improves greatly when we have the health to do the things we want to do. It is wise to say that healing yourself and others has a benefit not only on the individual, but on society as a whole.

When we experience trauma, say like a war, there is a great healing that takes place in the peace after it. We heal the soldiers. We heal the values of our nations. We even go so far as to heal ourselves.

On a more personal level when we are sick, we feel a great need to be healed. We want to feel better, to not be sick. Sometimes there is not time in our lives to do this. Perhaps we are stuck and do not know how to heal. Maybe medicine is working, yet only to an extent, and it is still not getting us to our personal goals of health.

When we take into account that Reiki is something that is addition to everything else in our lives, we begin to see it as an add-on to what we need. Let's explain that.

Say you're sick. You have decided to go into the hospital and they give you a diagnosis. You receive treatment. You begin to feel better.

Yet, you may still have blocked energies that were not addressed with your current healing. Reiki can step in and unblock those energies so that they can allow medicine to work faster or better.

That is how Reiki can truly benefit the physical. It is in addition to other disciplines that it functions at its highest ability, especially with those just beginning to learn and comprehend the power of Reiki energies. This is not to say that a true Reiki Master cannot heal with energies and power. They can. It is only a matter of practice and knowledge.

Consider someone who is sick, and who does not believe in energy work. The practicing Reiki master steps in and begins to work. Let's assume that the patient does not want to free energy, is afraid of the process and what is happening, they fear letting it flow through them. That is choice. They just want to be well. The Reiki Master has to work very hard in this case to help bring the energies in to properly effect a healing.

The mental side of health is where we can allow the Reiki Master in the same example as above to make healing progress much faster. When an individual is open to energies being moved around in their bodies, then the Reiki Master has less work to do to channel the energy to effect and heal to the issue at hand. Therefore, it allows for more healing with the same amount of energy as seen with the individual who does not want to flow, or is afraid to let it flow.

It is openness that makes Reiki so attractive and effective. When we begin to see how we are stuck or blocked mentally, spiritually, and energetically, we make much more progress so much more quickly. The flow of energies is not just a physical effect. Of course, flowing energies down and over a wounded spot on someone will make that spot feel better. Physical energy will even make the wound heal.

However, the true healing for the wounded is to put them into a place where they can heal themselves more effectively. This is the mental power of Reiki. When our energies flow around us in a smooth way, we relax and begin to feel like we can heal.

There is despair in being sick. There is fear in not knowing if we can get well again. When we have no tools to heal ourselves, except for outside sources, we begin to think the worst.

Reiki and its treatment allow all individuals involved to have the tools to work on themselves. Every Master learns from their students. Every artist learns from its subjects. This is the mental energies healing us all. When we flow, we can heal. When we heal, we improve life.

So, should everyone become a Reiki Master?

There are those who need help and those who can give help. It is proven that those who ask for help do not get as much mental benefit as for those who help others. The practitioner is just as likely to be healed as the patient is.

Becoming a Reiki Master and administering healing to others is not easily attained. The power for the recipient is in opening themselves for the Reiki practitioner to work energy healing on them. The power for the practitioner is that their healing energies will go far beyond their current patient.

It is the power of helping others where Reiki really shines. When you can heal another by unblocking them there is both a mental and the physical benefit. The lifestyle of the person you helped is amplified. Those around them will feel the effect as well.

We all have abilities, each and every one of us. It is just a matter of who and how we apply these abilities, that will bring about a more wonderful world.

The Energy Meridians of the Human Body

When the modality of Reiki was first developed by Mikao Usui, it was thought, and rightfully so, that the Reiki energy will flow to wherever it is needed. With the advent of knowledge shared between cultures and modalities, we have since discovered so much more of why the Reiki energy flows in the way that it does.

In part, it has to do with the energy centers within the body that we have now come to know as Chakras, and we will be getting to those in a moment. First, we will be discussing the actually energy lines that run through the body. In different cultures, they are known by different names. In the Chinese and Japanese healing modalities, they are known as vessels, or Meridians.

Interesting to note, science has actually discovered physical evidence of the Meridians in the body, now that our imaging systems have come far enough to measure them. There little tubular vessels that run through our body, directly where the corresponding Meridians have been known to ancient medicine techniques for centuries!

Just like the vascular system in our bodies, the energy has a natural flow in the way that it moves. Some move into the body, and some out. The main three lines move directly up and down the Chakra system. It is the Yin and Yang of energy movement through the body, and the Reiki energy naturally flows through the Meridians, down into the body and then back out again.

Reiki energy works intuitively, simply because it works directly with the energy centers and Meridians, because they connect directly with all physical aspects of the body, vascular, muscular, the endocrine system, the digestive system, etc. These energy systems, especially the energy centers at the Chakras, are also directly connected to our mental, emotional, and spiritual states of being, all which can directly affect our physical health and the energy that flows or stagnates in non-flow throughout our bodies.

By understanding more about the Meridians and the Chakras, even when working intuitively through the Reiki energy, we begin to have a better understanding of how it all works and how it all connects, which only deepens or connection to the Reiki energy and strengthens our ability to better utilize it when in need.

Within the human body, we have 12 pairs of major Meridians which run dually and symmetrically on either side of the body. These are the Heart, Lung, Spleen, Stomach, Kidney, Urinary Bladder, Small Intestine, Large Intestine, Thyroid (also called the Triple Warmer), Pericardium, Liver and Gall Bladder Meridians. I addition, there is a Governing and Central Meridian that run up the front and back side of the body between the mouth and pericardium.

Blockages, sluggishness, or malfunctions of these Meridians operate much like Chakras, where it disrupts the flow of energy, creating areas where illness, emotional damage, disrupted thinking, and other maladies can develop. By clearing these blockages and getting the energy moving again, we create pathways for the energy to flow to an ill-affected area and bring it back to health again.

Just knowing of the Meridians can help to better direct the energy when working with Reiki. Meridians don't flow in straight lines. They run through convoluted pathways that don't always make sense, except to the natural instincts and Divine Guidance of the Reiki energy itself. As you learn to intuitively feel where these energies flow to, you will start understanding the Meridians better, and that knowledge may help to better guide you when you feel the blockages present that can create the ill health your client may be experiencing.

Energy is all about flow and balance. When our energies are out of balance, or the flow disrupted, dependent upon where the disruption or imbalance takes place, it can cause issues with many different levels of our health and well-being. The Reiki energy hits these energy flows and starts them moving again, bringing your energy, and your health, back into balance.

Reiki and the 7 Chakras

Here is where Eastern medicine meets Indian medicine, for an amazing connection with healing energies. The Chakra system, an East Indian concept, is part of what the Reiki energy flows through when it is applying healing. Each one of the Chakras has corresponding points to our mental, emotional, and physical health.

By keeping the flow going through each of the Chakras, we keep the flow of energy moving that equates to good health. Starting with the lower Chakras, we get those moving first, because they are directly related to our basic, more instinctual energies that flow through our body. Once we get into the higher Chakras, we start awakening energies that can even further help guide the intuitive Reiki process, such as the Third Eye Chakra, which gives us knowledge beyond the physical senses... perfect for working with Reiki energy.

It is normal for one to actually work within themselves to clean out and open the Chakras, removing stagnant energy. This is the traditional Buddhist practice from centuries on. It is possible to work to help balance the flow in the Chakras of others, but great care must be taken. Often the blockages and stagnation when it comes to the Chakras goes far beyond the physical, with a basis in mental and emotional trauma. By clearing these Chakras without the individual you are working to heal being fully aware of what you are doing, you can open them up to past trauma which they may not be ready yet to deal with. This is why Chakra work through ancient teachings has always been a personal undertaking.

When working with the Chakras, whether for yourself or for others, there are different Reiki symbols for each of the seven Chakras, although the one used for the Third Eye and Crown Chakras are the same. Those symbols will be shown later in the chapter on Reiki symbols, so that you can have an understanding first of how symbols work before actually trying to use them out of context.

The other thing to understand when working with Chakras is that there are specific clues that the body can give you that will tell you specifically which Chakra is blocked, or disrupting the energy flow in a smooth manner. As you become more practiced in working with and reading the Reiki energy, listening to the Divine Guidance you receive during your healing sessions, you will better learn to identify what is going on before you even fully open yourself up.

There are actually more than seven Chakras, including ones in your hands that are used to guide the Reiki energy, and in your feet where the energy comes out of you to be grounded. Here, we will only be covering the seven main Chakras, as these are the ones that usually play with a direct correlation to the health and well-being of ourselves and others.

Starting from the root and working our way up to the Crown, there are seven basic Chakras. These are areas of energy within ourselves that can be activated, flowed, shielded, or examined.

Starting at the base of us, as is the growth of all life living on this planet, we look to the root first.

Muladhara (Root)

The *Muladhara* is located at the base of the spine. It is possible that the Root can be found a little bit lower. There is debate as to exact locations of Chakras. From traditional experience, they tend to be in similar locations, and yet not all humans are the same. So, we are looking at this Chakra as being in between the legs of an individual. Down at its base, down at the root of the core of the body.

This is a survival Chakra. It is also the location of our survival energies. When attacked, we curl into a ball and put our hands over our most vital spots, our *Muladhara*. Instinct tells us the root is our most important essential spot for survival.

The Root is a low-end grinding power. The ability to activate this Chakra connects us to the earth or others of our choosing. It can also be a grounding experience within ourselves. It is totally possible to ground ourselves to ourselves. This sounds like madness, however the Root does this for us. The *Muladhara,* when activated, can ground the person to not only the earth but themselves.

Muladhara inner state when active is a stillness. There is a great stability here. Imagine standing on rock versus sand. Or perhaps look at it as being planted into fertile soil versus sand. The *Muladhara* roots us into whatever we need. The more fertile we plant our roots the stronger they will be.

All Chakras are commonly related to a color. The color of the *Muladhara* is red. Red is the color of our blood, so it is only natural to associate it to our root. It is also one of the fastest frequency colors in our spectrum. The total light that humans see is red to violet. Red is one of the fastest colors we can see.

Here in lies a power of the *Muladhara*. Red moves swiftly and with assurance. With a little training, the *Muladhara* can allow a human body to accomplish almost anything, with power and swiftness.

Activation of this Chakra comes from the mantra, *I am*. The *Muladhara* defines us. Our roots are who we are. The Root Chakra is who we are. Chanting or meditation on the words, *I am*, and focusing on the energies located between our legs will charge up the Root and make it go. *I am*.

This is a red glow. When actively concentrating on the *I am*, the *Muladhara* takes fear to calm fear. Actually, it goes all the way to control fear. Imagine life-threatening fear. And now concentrate on what can make you survive the most from your life ending. The best Chakra to access at this point is the red glow of the Root. We will drop into a place where we can be grounded and survive even with our worst fears.

This is the Chakra that increases overall health as well. It is the place of starting healing for all of us. Many will say that the head and mind are the key. Indeed, they are. Mental health is very beneficial. It is when we look at where we get our healing power, we see it starts with our Root.

Grounding is a way to calm and connect. The *Muladhara*, when it thumps nice and slow, accomplishes a great focusing. It is a centering on anything we choose to concentrate on. This is the grounding and the starting point of all healing. When we utilize our Root Chakra, we can accomplish almost anything in a very primal way of sophisticated duration.

Svadhisthana (Sacral)

The *Svadhisthana* is located right around where a woman's womb is. The lower abdomen is also considered a location of this Chakra. Some will say a location like genitals is where the Sacral Chakra resides, however it is debatable that this may be a bit too low on the human body. Concentration on the lower abdomen is most likely a good starting point to find the location of the Sacral Chakra.

This Chakra is often associated with desire. The wanting of something, anything for that matter, is the purpose of the Sacral. The *Svadhisthana* is often associated with sexual desire and pleasure and procreation. It is the desire for almost anything that can drive us to action, sexual or not. The Sacral accomplishes desire, and desire is best as a wanting. We want this and that.

*Svadhisthana*s' inner state is one of tears. Tears of joy or anguish can be found here. This is to say that this Chakra is one of emotions. When active, and doing what it does, the *Svadhisthana* is almost pure emotion. Imagine the joy of a baby born, or feel the guts ripped out of you when you lose someone you love. The Sacral is the emotion Chakra.

Its color is orange. When we draw a sun, we draw it with orange and yellow. It is not the purity of the yellow solar plexus, but a blend of the red Root Chakra and the willingness of the yellow Solar

Plexus Chakra. Orange is also a color associated with speed. It is relatively quick on the color spectrum. Emotions can be quick. Remember a nice orange glow when activating this Chakra, and it can yield swift emotional response to whatever you are focused on.

Meditation on *I feel* will activate the *Svadhisthana*. When we concentrate on our feelings and that we have them, they can drive us in ways that logic does not comprehend. *I feel*, is that we are beings that have feelings. For example, depression can indeed cause us to curl up into a ball and feel like dying. The end result of removing judgment from feelings, makes it so that feelings drive us to take action to make it so we eventually do not get as depressed as we once were. *I feel*. It affects me. I change. I feel is a state of being, not to be judged.

Sexuality is said to reside with the Sacral Chakra. Some do debate that the root is our true sexual Chakra. When the *Svadhisthana* is discussed it is associated with the desire of sex, not necessarily the act itself. The Sacral is a Chakra is mostly about the desire to procreate, whereas the Root is about the actual act. This *Svadhisthana* emotional response to our biological urge to procreate is one of sexual vitality, and then we have feelings.

This orange Chakra is a fire Chakra. This fire leads to our physical powers. Imagine a great bonfire burning a bright orange. Jumping into that fire will incinerate us. The Sacral Chakra allows the power of something so destructive as orange fire to be access and worked with in a safe way.

The *Svadhisthana* energizes us. It is not necessarily giving us energy; it is causing us to charge up to make us go. Yes, any of our Chakras can be utilized to produce energy, however the Sacral is the emotion and desire charging all other Chakras. It is the core of thought and feelings as to where our energies come from. We feel and then we are energized to action.

Manipura **(Solar Plexus)**

The *Manipura* is located above the navel. Remember to consider that the human body is not a piece of paper but a shape with volume and mass. Our Solar Plexus is in our centers and is unique to each, because we all have the same body in theory only. A passing of a hand over the *Manipura* will allow you to see where it is. Above the belly button and below the sternum is the best place to start.

This Chakra is a place of willingness. Will, and our will, takes a great center focus when we activate the *Manipura*. It is beneficial to remember that our will is a twofold concept. There is a willingness and a willfulness. Willfulness is when we say nope, not doing that. Willingness is openness to action, even if we do not act. When we are working with the *Manipura* we are working with our will to do anything. How we approach that work is up to us, open and willing or in a state of being willful and not.

The inner state of the *Manipura* is one of laughter and joy. It is also one of anger and aggression. This tells us that when we enter this Chakra, we are getting ready to work. Laughter leads us to more laughter. The will to gain more laughter is the core of the Solar. Anger also leads us to action. These inner states of being promote action. This is a work Chakra.

The color of the *Manipura* is yellow. In the East, yellow is the color of the champion. In the West it is the color of the sun. Yellow tends to be a color of joy and happiness. Yellow is also the caution tape of all workplaces. A nice yellow glow is a great way to keep working all day long, nice and safe.

I do, is the meditation that starts up this Chakra. *I do* this and *I do* that, is the battle cry of the *Manipura*. When we have the willingness to really charge up our yellow Chakra, we can slow down the pulses of it, and give a nice slow grind, with any work we choose. Eventually this Chakra takes over and work becomes something of a treat versus a chore. For we get energies back from ourselves when we meditate on, *I do*.

The *Manipura* calms emotions. Considering how close it is to the *Svadhisthana* these two Chakras can work in concert. The feelings and emotions created by the Sacral can be calmed down by the Solar. In the doing of anything, the emotions originally causing work, are calmed and satisfied. This also works with frustrations. When we are frustrated, we can remove frustration by calming our emotions and putting in a little bit of, *I do* into action.

This is also a fire Chakra. It is an energizing Chakra. It is a slow yellow burn that lasts us all through our work. This is not necessarily physical work. This can be utilized to the higher mental work of the upper Chakras. Connection of the *Manipura* to any Chakra will cause it to maneuver from a place of idle, to a place of actual doing.

Anahata (Heart)

The *Anahata* is located in the center of the chest. An anatomical heart is located a little lower and to the left of this, in ourselves. Lower and to the right when facing another. The *Anahata* is very often found as an energy radiating from the center of our chests.

This is the love Chakra. Love has so many different conceptual definitions that it can be everything from actual physical love, to the universal understanding. No matter how we look at it, love is rarely selfish and is often in the benefit of others. When we love ourselves, we experience this benefit firsthand. It is the love of everything that the *Anahata* can inspire love in us all.

Heart Chakra, our inner state of being, is one of compassion. As Buddha sat in compassion for the world, he was in a Heart Chakra. When we utilize this Chakra for its fullest potential, we begin to see that there is a compassion needed for everyone and everything around us. It is not just a metaphorical wisdom here. There is a lot to be said for loving everyone and everything.

The color of the *Anahata* is green. Green is the color of plant life and we often associate the color of the world to green. In fact, from space, Earth is a blue marble. Down here, where we all live, green is color of life and growth. It is interesting that we paint our hearts for valentine's day with a red and not a green. The Heart Chakra is green.

I love, is the meditation on this energy. When we concentrate on nothing but, *I love*, we begin to see the world around us in a new light. There is a love that already exists that we can touch and see. When we live in a place of love we live in a place of bliss. As long as we remind ourselves that we are still rooted creatures, it is best for us to remain in a place of love.

The balance of this Chakra leads to circulatory wellness. This is the systems of the physical heart that these energies can heal and work with. Blood flows, and the quality of this blood stems directly to the *Anahata*. Consider a green light when we look at our blood flowing through our veins. That balance of love can lead to great health benefits.

To be more precise, this is a spiritual love. The source of it comes from us understanding what love is in a universal oneness. In other words, there is a great pattern among all life and we all touch it. It is when we touch it with love powering ourselves, we begin to see a real reason to be here.

This is the first water connection we have to a Chakra. Water flowing like a well gushing out and over its walls, is an excellent meditation on the *Anahata*. It is a calming water. One drink, soothes and relaxes us.

Universal Oneness and love, spiritually calming and soothing ourselves and others, this is the way of the Heart.

Vishddha (Throat)

The *Vishddha* is located in the throat. This may be the closest you will get to any of the seven Chakras. Even the Chakras connected to our heads are a little more difficult to find. When we touch our throats and the throats of others, we are touching the *Vishddha*, almost directly.

When we consider how close we can get to this Chakra we begin to see its value. It is a communication energy. It is not always about speech. In fact, the *Vishddha* is a place of creative expressions. Communication is so much more than just speaking. There is a subtly here. Most access the *Vishddha*, speak, and are done. When we take time to look at what communication really is, we see that it has a complexity that can be quickly overlooked with just words.

The *Vishddha* is a place of creativity. We create when we communicate. Think about two people who do not speak the same language. How will they communicate? The Throat Chakra steps in with its creativity and transverses a solution.

This is the inner state of the Throat Chakra. It is the synthesizing of ideas into symbols. Considering that Reiki takes quite a bit of symbol to work, and that the *Vishddha* is a birthplace of those symbols.

This inner state of being and taking time to formulate image and symbol from our own source can be daunting at first. Say we are only good at drawing stick figures. This is ok. The Throat Chakra works with what we have. Even if it is crayons.

The color of this Chakra is bright blue. This is the color of the day sky. The color of the blue sea. The bright blue is one of communication again. When we communicate, we often see it as a blue light. There is something to be said in the fact that most of the communication company logos of our time, are light blue in color.

I speak, is the meditation here. Remember that we have two ears and only one mouth, therefore a great leader listens twice as much as they speak. This is a true form of communication. *I speak*, is not always about voicing opinion or talking over another. *I speak*, is a meditation showing us that we do have the ability to speak and that it is a communication tool. Listening is also. *I speak* charges up the *Vishddha* for all forms of communication.

Once again, we are connecting water to water. The *Vishddha* is a water Chakra. And once again, we get the same benefits from true water communication. It calms, soothes and relaxes us and others around us.

When we speak with a true voice of the *Vishddha,* we find that others around us calm down and listen.

Ajna (Third Eye)

Ajna is located in the center of the forehead. The Third Eye is just above your other two eyes. In between the eyebrows, is often where it is found. It is a touch of the middle of your forehead.

Ajna is the Chakra of seeing. Considering it is literally referred to as an eye, we can use it to see more clearly, as well as having a fresh perspective. It is not a place of understanding. This is where Chakra connections gets a little difficult. *Ajna* is not understanding. *Ajna* is seeing. Seeing is observation mostly. Very little is done with the

Third Eye other than to see the universe for what it is.

And therein lies its true power. It is intuition that *Ajna* really promotes. Intuition is a combination of two things. Feelings and logic make up intuition. When we observe with *Ajna* and see anything for what it is, two things happen inside us. We logically figure out what we are observing, and second, we have a feeling in ourselves. It is somewhere in between that the Third Eye operates. A wisdom, so to speak, about logically and emotionally observing. Intuition is the result of the Third Eye.

The inner state of *Ajna* is knowing. Knowing is very different from understanding. An example that may hit closer to home is, knowing a pattern is very different from understanding a pattern. The Third Eye knows only. It is when we administer our own agenda on top of what we think we know that the Third Eye loses its perspective. Considering seeing is mostly about perspective, the eye is lost when we inundate ourselves. It is best to not have personal agenda perspective when working with *Ajna*, to let the ego go.

The color of the Third Eye is indigo. Dark deep rich purple is a color not found in nature often. This is the rarity of *Ajna*. It is the color of royals and a color coveted by artists.

Considering violet and indigo are some of the slowest colors in our visual spectrum, allowing slow movements with Third Eye may be beneficial. Consider allowing purple to go slow like it does in nature.

I see, is the chant for *Ajna*. It is very difficult to remove all thoughts and agendas and opinions when we just see anything. The being of, I see, is a state of being visual only. A place where we can just relax and see the universe for what it is. When we relax our Third Eye, it sees all manners of energies.

The balance of *Ajna* leads to a psychic perception as well. Belief in psychic abilities or not, we are talking about seeing them. It is here where we perceive auras and energies that we do not see with our normal eyes. The abilities of psychic individuals are founded here. The Third Eye opens and sees, yet does not judge.

This Chakra is an air Chakra. One of aloofness and necessary solo, alone time. It is difficult to share your Third Eye with another. Opening another's Third Eye is incredibly rash and dangerous. There are some things that we are not ready to see. This is the soaring of air. The wearing down of mountains and whipping the oceans into a thundering hurricane.

Ajna is a meditative place. Third Eye will not function under non meditative states. Distractions of life can impede the work done by the Third Eye. This is the way and the why, gurus spend so much time solo.

It is best to be reminded in that *Ajna* is a promoter of the birthplace of intuition. We are not to take direct action from our Third Eye without much examination. It is designed to reflect back inside of us to see what is happening, and then we can solely observe.

Sahasrara (Crown)

The *Sahasrara* is located top of head. It is often seen as a giant lotus flower on top of our skulls. This is to say that the Crown Chakra is, and may not necessarily be, within our forms. It may indeed hover a little over us. Individuals vary.

This is the Chakra of understanding. When we come up from our Root into our work, then up to our hearts, promoting communication, and then observing, we eventually come to understanding. This is the place of the Crown. What is it to understand something completely? That is the question the *Sahasrara* answers. It is only when we fully understand anything that we are actually just scratching the surface of our crowns existence.

The inner state of *Sahasrara* is a state of bliss. Imagine the ability to understand something fully. There is an exercise about a thousand petal lotus.

Each petal unique. On top of that each petal is its own color. Sitting and contemplating this lotus to a full understanding of each petal and its overall purpose, is bliss. At least some say it is.

We are in the color of violet. The top of the color spectrum. The slowest of frequencies. Indeed, the *Sahasrara* requires an immense amount of time to not only activate but to use for understanding. Some do not accomplish this in an entire lifetime. Violet light, shining from a multicolored lotus flower, this is the color of the Crown.

I understand, is the slow and painful way to meditate on the *Sahasrara*. When we think we have understood whatever we are working on, we then break and come back to it again, and find that we missed something. *I understand* is also a state of being. We do not understand until we are open to understanding. It is only when we open our minds and allow for almost all information and energies to be observed, do we actually, fully, understand.

This Chakra when turned on has quite a few more benefits other than understanding. When understanding finds balance, there is a vitality to the mind. This can even go so far as to make it so that those who ignite and meditate on the Crown can develop psychic abilities.

We are still in a place of air, rushing around and always floating. We are easily brushed harshly, when we fly. The currents of air play much more abruptly than the currents of water. Consider standing next to that thousand petal lotus, then consider floating above it... this is why it is so difficult to understand.

This is the Chakra that promotes the most thought. It requires an immense amount of thought to even understand the most basic things in this universe. Considering those who say they know it all, that is saying that you have mastered the Crown, therefore mastered the knowledge of the universe itself.

The *Sahasrara* is a Chakra that can see the universal patterns and understand them. With the limitless expanse of our existence, the Crown is unlimited as well. Therefore, we are unlimited when we meditate on the concept of, I understand, even when we do not quite have it yet.

Chapter 3: Reiki Symbols

You will find that many of the Reiki Masters, especially those trained in the more traditional styles, find the symbols as sacred, and not to be shared with the uninitiated, or in this case, unattuned. And rightfully so. Using the Reiki energy is not something that should be undertaken by those who are unaware of its power or nature. Even Reiki practitioners are not taught the use of symbols until they are initiated for the level of Reiki 2.

It is not as relevant these days, as the free flow of information in books and the internet allows for people to look up the Reiki symbols for themselves. For the most part, the Reiki symbols are said to have little or no energy use value in and of themselves. There have been experiments that have demonstrated that without the initiation at the beginning of a Reiki level, that even students with intuitive abilities have had little success achieving consistent and powerful use of the Reiki symbols. The attunement at the end of a Reiki level even further strengthens this ability, as its "sets" the symbol into your own energy for instant recall.

That being said, it is possible, with work and dedication, to achieve your own mastery levels through Reiki. It is a lot of work and dedication! Look at how many years it took Usui, the originator of Reiki, to find the power of these special symbols, and he was specifically seeking an energetic healing method. So yes, it is possible to work toward attuning yourself to the symbols. Be prepared to devote yourself to the practices you have learned within this book, and the seeking of Divine Guidance from without, in order to achieve your own special connection to the Reiki symbols and their energy.

Think of the Reiki symbols as keys that unlock the energy connection and guidance of your higher mind. After attunement, you are able to use them more like buttons, to gain instant results. They do not physically have to be drawn in the air or on the subject for which you would use them, they can instead be visualized, and the power is just as amazing and potent.

Keep in mind that practice makes perfect, and the drawing of the symbols in the air (usually done with your index finger), helps to set their shape, form, and energy in your mind so that you can better recall them in a visual fashion, if that is how you choose to work with the Reiki symbols.

Also keep in mind, as with any energy work, working with Reiki energy is both an intuitive and personal experience. As you connect more strongly and work with understanding the Reiki energy, you will find yourself changing and adapting how you work with it to best suit yourself.

So, in essence, there is no true right or wrong way to work with the energy, or the Divine Guidance that you are given when connected to the Reiki energy. You may find yourself developing entirely new symbols or ways of working with Reiki energy. You may find that drawing the symbols with your thumb works better for you than your index finger.

Whatever the way you work with the Reiki energy, it is important to keep in mind that your dedication and daily practice only strengthens your connection to both the energy and to Divine Guidance, so dedicate yourself to spending daily time, if you can, and you will find that amazing things will unfold in your life.

About the Reiki Symbols

There are three primary Reiki symbols that are taught when students are initiated into Reiki level 2. The fourth symbol is taught to those who gain Master level in Reiki, and the fifth symbol is used by those who are Masters to attune the symbols into other initiates.

The symbols themselves are based on an old version of the Kanji system of Japanese writing, but also hold ties to ancient Sanskrit symbols. Their power is very old, much older than the initial 140+ years since Usui first develop the modality that we know as Reiki today. There are now more than just these original 5 symbols developed and taught by Mikao Usui. But there are far too many to list them all here and do them justice. Instead, we will be focusing on those original 5 symbols.

The Original Reiki Symbols and Meanings

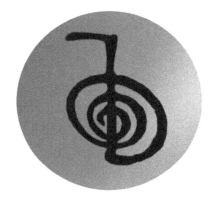

Cho Ku Rei

This is the Reiki power symbol. The swirl with a strike through the middle implies contemplation with decision. It is an opening and closing symbol. What is meant by this symbol is that it can be used to start up and close down energy work.

Cho Ku Rei is not just about being a door of power. It is a placement holder. It puts all the powers of the Universe into the spiral allowing the practitioner to follow the energies to be accessible for what they need.

It has a primary use, and that is to boost Reiki power. When used, consider a door. The more you open the door the more light gets in. The more you close the door the more light stays out. This is the way of the *Cho Ku Rei*. It is one of volume and transfer of Reiki energy.

Since it is referred to as a door, we can use it to connect to the Reiki energy in that way. It is the way to start a session. Some even go so far as to draw the symbol on their hands so that the energies can come straight into other Reiki symbols and therefore out of their hands.

It is a way to seal a session at the end. *Cho Ku Rei* can be utilized in a way to capture energies that are extra so that nothing behind remains. Leftover energies may have an effect that the practitioner did not intend. When the *Cho Ku Rei* is used at the end of a session, the energies collect back into it and dissipate along the spiral.

It is a way to empower the hands and collect energies back in. It is up to the Master to open the door and allow those energies to expel back into the Universe.

It is often a practice to run this symbol over the Chakras of the individual practicing. It is not only used to charge up the hands, it can also be used to open a door or two of the Chakras that may need to be used.

This is a symbol that empowers the other Reiki symbols. What is meant by this, is that when a symbol is created this symbol can activate, empower and shut down other symbols. It is best to start here.

The *Cho Ku Rei* does have more of a practical function. It very much helps spot treatments. It is a collector of information. When we understand how to read that information, we can begin to see what needs to be treated.

This symbol also clears negative energies. Since it represents a spiral, that spiral can spin both ways. One way to spin is to pull in negative energies, the other direction will expel them out. Rotation of symbols and animation of symbols is a style all its own.

Cho Ku Rei is a protection symbol. Once again, we look at a door. When you close that door and lock it, you are keeping out or holding in materials and energy. We can indeed barricade behind our *Cho Ku Rei*.

When this symbol is passed over food, it makes meals more nutritious and healthier.

This is a symbol of energizing and activation. When we take medication, the *Cho Ku Rei* can accent the effectiveness of that medication. It can even reduce the side effects of modern medicine. The spiral is one of addition to more than its own power.

The *Cho Ku Rei* also improves relationships. Imagine taking the time to contemplate someone else's spiral, and then coming to a decisive point with them. Since the *Cho Ku Rei* collects information and then shares it, that is a communication tool that all relationships could use.

This examination and collection of information leads to less provocations and more understanding in the laws of attraction. Instinctively, we understand what we are attracted to. The *Cho Ku Rei* allows us to take our time in the spiral and examine what is actually going on, then take decisive action to achieve it.

The power symbol is used in many different ways. Remember that style is unique to all who use this symbol. Activation of *Cho Ku Rei* will start, stop, or add to any other energy work being done.

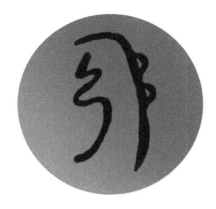

Sei He Ki

The *Sei He Ki* is a symbol of mental and emotional healing. Mental blocks happen most often when we become ill, or can even cause illness, and this symbol can assist with that.

Sei He Ki traditionally means where the Earth and sky meet. We consider this to be the horizon, however, we need to think of it more like the sky and Earth merging. When we have both power of air and earth combined, we become a controlled mountain.

It is also traditionally a symbol of the Universe and man becoming one. This may be left to the theologians of our time. It is said that emotions combined with a little logic leads to universal understanding. The *Sei He Ki* is a combination symbol.

Different practitioners use this symbol in different ways. One example is to draw the *Cho Ku Rei* that connects to source. Then follow by drawing the *Sei He Ki* symbol over the troubled area. This will allow Earth and sky to meet, and bring forth the energies needed to help emotional flow.

Remember to close with *Cho Ku Rei*.

When *Cho Ku Rei* is used to stabilize, the *Sei He Ki* effects of this symbol are sustained over time.

This is the memory power symbol. It is used in many different ways, including getting rid of habits and addictions, and even going so far as to improve relationships.

Sei He Ki empowers affirmations. When we state we want to do something, *Sei He Ki* can be used to empower that statement. It is in the doing that this symbol truly shines, because emotions tell us how to act, when we listen properly to ourselves.

This symbol represents a personal bodyguard. One that protects not just our physical form, but a place to entrust our emotions, and know that they will be provided for. It is also a protector for those who are receiving as well.

There are many different ways this symbol has practicality. For example, the *Sei He Ki* is used to lessen headaches.

On the other side of the physical, to more of a metaphysical state of being, the *Sei He Ki* can find your lost car keys.

This is because this symbol is the synchronization of harmony and everything in nature.

When we connect to everything natural with the *Sei He Ki*, we begin to gain a much more positive outlook. Life becomes and remains happier.

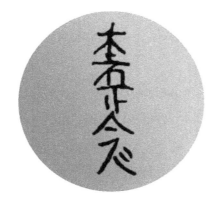

Hon Sha Ze Sho Nen

This is the Reiki distance symbol. It is used to heal from afar, or when the individual you are working for is not comfortable with touch.

Due to its traditional sense of having no present, past or future, the *Hon Sha Ze Sho Nen* is, and requires, a personal style.

Some are attuned to close quarters healing. Others can and do healing from afar. As long as permission is given, *Hon Sha Ze Sho Nen*, when used and activated, can cover great distances.

One example is to activate the *Cho Ku Rei* power symbol. Then write the person's name and/or or the issues that are occurring on paper and hold it.

Draw *Hon Sha Ze Sho Nen* in the air above the paper three times.

Repeat the individual's name or issues at hand more than once.

Draw the *Cho Ku Rei* again to close.

The *Hon Sha Ze Sho Nen* allows the input and output of positive energies just about anywhere, very quickly and easily. This is not a beginner symbol, but one of more advanced work. Its simplicity makes it so anyone can target energies at range. Remember the slow wisdom of the *Cho Ku Rei* power symbol and always attach it to ranged energy work.

The *Hon Sha Ze Sho Nen* is very popular with those who are uncomfortable with being touched.

We are talking about a spirit of harmony here. The *Hon Sha Ze Sho Nen* is an energy that can heal the past, as well as send energy into the future. It is a healing that does not require much direct work. In that way, the *Hon Sha Ze Sho Nen* is a symbol that can heal independently on its own.

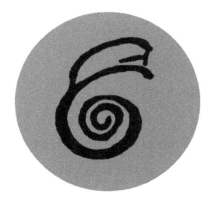

Dai Ko Myo

The *Dai Ko Myo* is the master symbol. It is a symbol of great enlightenment, and is often referred to as the bright shining light.

This symbol can be activated in many different ways. The most common is to draw it with your palm center. Then, giving a little time to visualize it, it allows the *Dia Ko Myo* the ability to manifest. Drawing the symbol with your finger will bring it even more into form. Spending time to draw *Dai Ko Myo* with your Third Eye will allow sight and wisdom and intuition to reside inside the symbol.

The *Dai Ko Myo* is the channel opening attunement. This is a very powerful symbol. The energies transferred here are some of the highest and most potent in Reiki practice.

The *Dai Ko Myo* is mostly used to heal locations and powers such as Chakras and auras. This symbol is also used to heal the subconscious. There is much mental work done here. Considering how the *Ajna* Third Eye functions, *Dia Ko Myo* is a symbol of intuition, as well as one of gathering knowledge.

The *Dai Ko Myo* is a symbol that draws out negative energy from the individual and allows the individual to dissipates it.

The *Dai Ko Myo* is a symbol that develops personal growth as well. It is a symbol of self-awareness. The

Dia Ko Myo is best utilized for spiritual development. This is the placement of the *Ajna*. It is the placement of intuition. It is the symbol of not only seeing what is, it is understanding it as well.

The *Dai Ko Myo*, with its purification ability, is often used as a symbol to charge and clear crystals. Crystals can store mas amounts of patterns. The *Dai Ko Myo* is used to channel out this material so that crystals can be empty for new attunement.

This symbol is a symbol that can be drawn to improve immunity. When the body gets blocked in an energy fashion, the *Dai Ko Myo* allows energy flow all through the body.

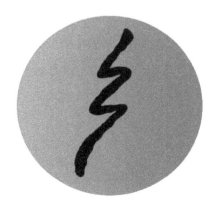

Raku

Raku is a symbol mostly used for attunement. This is the symbol used when a new practitioner is created in Reiki.

Raku is known as the lightning bolt. Considering how lightning works, this is a very accurate symbol for us to begin with. A lightning strike does not come from the sky. The sky calls upon energies and the earth answers. Energy jumps from the Earth into the sky, and then crashes back down to Earth in a place of dissipation.

Raku is a brilliant way to define what Reiki does. The cycle created by all energy work and symbols is one of a circular nature. Up and down, in and out, no matter how you describe what Reiki is, and its symbols do, it is a good reminder to consider that we are working with circles.

Raku banks the fire. What we mean by this is that charges the energy.

Raku is also a style of glazed ceramic firing. Taking this example, we can begin to see how the give and take of the *Raku* symbol works. When we low fire ourselves with a beautiful gasoline glaze, we are in a place of the practice of Reiki. We come about more beautiful than when we started.

The *Raku* symbol is one of attunement. Solid purification of the Universal Life Force is flowed into and through the lightning bolt.

When used as a grounding tool, one only needs to consider the lightning bolt.

Crystal Work with Reiki

Using crystals in your Reiki session when healing yourself or someone else, is one of the non-traditional styles of Reiki energy use that we listed earlier. Most practitioners who use crystals with their Reiki energy do so to directly work with the Chakras, and unblocking the energy flows. They choose stones when guided to do so, and use them for the healing benefit of the individual with whom they are working.

Stones used for Reiki are often given an attunement all of their own, sometimes prior to each use by the Reiki practitioner. Sometimes the Reiki practitioner will inscribe the power of a particular Reiki symbol to enhance the work they are already doing.

Divine Guidance is the key to working with crystals and combining them with the Reiki energy. Every crystal and stone have their own individual energy resonance, and it works to add another layer and combine the energy with that already brought into the session by the Reiki practitioner.

As mentioned before, there is no right or wrong way to work with the Reiki energy. Although, it should be said that the one less beneficial way to is let your ego get in the way and make decisions on how to use the energy without Divine Guidance. Listen to that voice from within, allow it to guide you as to whether or not you should use crystals or stones in your Reiki practice, and as to how you should utilize them for the highest and greatest good of yourself and those on whom you work.

With that in mind, here are some of the more commonly used crystals and stones for working with healing energy.

Clear Seed Crystals: Clear Seed Crystals are clear and thin with smooth sides. The more clarity it has, the more powerful it is to work with. They help to better connect us to the Reiki energy, and to one another. Clear Seed Crystal are clear, and are particularly open and suited to the imprint of energies for future use.

Amethyst: Amethyst is well-known for its powers of protection, especially from negative energies and thoughts. It also resonates with and expands the higher mind, better opening you for connection to the source of Reiki and Divine Inspiration and Guidance. It is often use in Reiki Crystal energy work to connect to the Crown Chakra.

Selenite: Selenite has the rare property among crystals to not only cleanse and purify, but is never in need of cleansing or purification for itself. It recharges itself, which makes it extremely suitable and connected to the Reiki energies.

Celestite: Celestite helps to reduce stress and bring about a state of relaxation, which is always optimal for healing. It also helps to connect you to your higher states of mind.

Citrine: Citrine aids in adjusting and adapting to change, which can be essential when working with the Reiki energies. It also helps to open your mind to Divine Guidance and intuition.

Fluorite: Fluorite can be extremely beneficial in spiritual awakening, and allows the work and flow of large amounts of energy.

Labradorite: Labradorite aids in elevating your levels of conscious awareness and your connection to the Universal Source of Life Force energy.

Lapis Lazuli: Lapis Lazuli is a stone used for centuries to aid in meditation, and for trance work and working in other forms of altered states of consciousness.

Moldavite: Moldavite works well to help balance the energies of both you and your client. It promotes healing, and connects you to your higher self and to helps you to be more receptive to Divine Guidance and communication.

Opal: Opal aids in connecting to altered states of consciousness, and allows for energy absorption.

Peridot: Peridot allows you to be more receptive to higher aspects of information.

Quartz: Quartz is a "go to" stone/crystal for many energy workers. It channels and amplifies large amounts of energy, promotes healing, and better opens you to Divine Guidance.

Rhodochrosite: Rhodochrosite aids in connecting the subconscious with the conscious, and works well as an energy transmitter.

Sapphire: Sapphire is an incredible stone for tapping into and sending energy, as well as helping to receive and interpret Divine Guidance.

In addition to Reiki energy work with stones or crystals, here is a list of stones generally used to connect with the Chakras for aiding in clearing and balancing the energy channels:

Root Chakra: For the Root Chakra, any stone or crystal that is red will usually connect and resonate with this base energy, such as jasper, carnelian, fire agate, bloodstone, etc.

Sacral Chakra: For the Sacral Chakra, any stone or crystal that is orange will usually connect and resonate with this center's energy, such as jasper, fire agate, carnelian, sunstone, etc.

Solar Plexus Chakra: For the Solar Plexus Chakra, any stone or crystal that is yellow will usually connect and resonate with this center's energy, such as amber, citrine, tiger's eye, etc.

Heart Chakra: For the Heart Chakra, any stone or crystal that is green will usually connect and resonate with this center's energy, such as jade, chrysocolla, malachite, emerald, prehnite, green fluorite, etc. Rose Quartz, even though pink in color, is also very powerful crystal for working with the Heart Chakra. Some schools of thoughts involving Chakras actually use pink in place of green for the Heart Chakra.

Throat Chakra: For the Throat Chakra, any stone or crystal that is blue will usually connect and resonate with this center's energy, such as aquamarine, lapis lazuli, larimar, tanzanite, azurite, etc.

Third Eye Chakra: For the Third Eye Chakra, any stone or crystal that is indigo will usually connect and resonate with this center's energy, such as labradorite, lapis lazuli, kyanite, amethyst, etc.

Crown Chakra: For the Crown Chakra, it is not so much a color that connects, but it is more any stone or crystal that is of a high energy nature will usually connect and resonate with this center's energy, such as amethyst, labradorite, selenite, danburite, charolite, nuummite, etc.

As previously stated, don't choose the crystals or stones for your Reiki sessions based on their properties. These were included to help give you a better understanding of why the stone might be chosen. Sometimes this knowledge can help aid you in better connecting to the energy and affect a better healing.

Allow the Reiki energy and Divine Guidance tell you what stone should be used, how you should use it, or whether it should be used at all. Reiki is an intuitive process, and you need to be open to Divine Guidance to help heal for the highest and greatest benefit of what you are trying to accomplish for yourself and for others.

Chapter 4: Reiki Healing

We've discussed Reiki origins, what it is, and what Reiki energy is. There are many different styles of healing out there, from Western medicine to acupuncture, therapy, and many, many forms of energy healing. So why Reiki?

What is the Difference Between Reiki and Other Energy Healing?

On the surface, from someone taking an outside look at different forms of energy healing, including that of spiritual energy healing, Reiki looks to be the same as any of the others. Even some of the more non-traditional Reiki forms have become more of an energy healing that incorporates elements of Reiki, rather than pure Reiki itself.

There are differences between the different energy healing modalities and each other, Reiki included. It is the same source of energy used by all of them, although sometimes given different names and attributes. The true difference between all of the energy healing, Reiki included, is in how the practitioner connects to or receives the energy, and in how they ultimately use it for healing.

In essence, when properly used, they will all get you to the same result, it is just how you get there, and sometimes, how quickly you arrive at your chosen destination.

Most energy forms of healing use the hands, either through touch or pure channel to send or transmit the energies being used for the healing process. Some use the heart as the focus for their channel. Some use the Chakras, although even with the Chakras, there are smaller energy centers noted in the palms and feet which are sometimes used for channeling the Chakra energy for healing.

The biggest difference between Reiki and other energy systems used for healing, is the use of symbols. Obviously, the origins of each of the systems have differences, and how they connect with the energy and how they use it to treat someone in a healing session also varies.

In most types of energy healing, and outside source is called upon to provide the energy and channel that healing through the practitioner. In most of these cases, it is Universal Life Force energy, although it may be called by different names.

In all cases, the practitioner used themselves as a channel for the energy, a conduit of sorts. Almost none of them use their own personal energy. They would not be able to effectively treat numbers of people without replenishing the original source of energy from within themselves. That is not effective healing for anyone.

With some of the more modernized, non-traditional forms of Reiki, the attunement process may not be sufficient enough to deal with the release of some of the emotions that may arise when energy centers are unblocked for flow. This even includes the attunement with the emotional symbols.

Many times, these attunements and teachings are done over a weekend, which is not enough to delve into the many emotional situations that can arise within a client when their energy becomes unblocked and starts to flow. Reiki Masters who spend time in contemplation of the higher aspects of the mind and with the Reiki energies often are better capable of handling these emotional situations from a place of higher understanding.

Other energy practitioners learn to heal by practicing their methods of connecting to and drawing upon the energy source. Those who work with Reiki tune their consciousness into the energy through the use of the Reiki symbols, which then connects them to the source of energy. Regardless of the practice, they all work with the human energy field that surrounds and resides within the body, and channel the energy into that field to affect a healing.

No matter the form of energy healing, Reiki or otherwise, energy healing is beneficial to others, and to yourself, especially when used for the highest and greatest good. With any energy healing, it should not be a substitute for traditional medicine forms of treatment and/or care. Reiki and other energy healing modalities may indeed produce better, and possibly even full healing results. However, most practitioners are not at that level of full healing capability, and their energy work can enhance and speed up the results are being worked upon through traditional/allopathic medicine practices.

Preparing Yourself

Preparing yourself for working with Reiki is an on-going process. Yes, there are the smaller steps of preparing yourself for a Reiki treatment, preparing yourself for a Reiki initiation and class, or preparing yourself for a Reiki attunement to move up in levels of mastery until you achieve the level of Master and teacher.

We've already discussed preparing yourself for a Reiki session for the healing of yourself or others, through the use of *Gassho*. This is a very important step in focusing on, calling in, and working with the Reiki energies.

If you truly want to work with the Reiki energies and make it part of your life, there are further preparations that you can do, for your mental, emotional, and physical sides of yourself, that can better open, and keep open, your channels to get the highest and greatest benefit for yourself and others.

Preparing yourself in this case, is learning to live a lifestyle that keeps your body healthy and in tune with the Universal Life Force so that you become better connected, in all aspects of your life. It is living for the health of yourself, so that you may better facilitate the healing of others.

It is also keeping yourself clean as a conduit for the Universal Life Force and more open to Divine intuition and guidance. This a natural way of living that allows you to connect to everything and observe it is a whole, a completeness. You no longer look at illness in the various levels of health and see it as individual issues to be healed, you learn to see the entire picture and acknowledge the other things around the illness or sickness that may be contributing to the problem of poor health.

Illness manifested in the physical does not always have a root cause in the physical. Sometimes its emotional, psychological, spiritual. By preparing yourself to live in the moment, to live holistically, you are always prepared to connect to the energy and see what the true root cause is, and you allow for Divine Guidance to come in and address the root of what needs to be healed, rather than just staying at the surface. We do this by allowing ourselves to live holistically, so that we may experience holistically.

Part of the basis of *Gassho*, when preparing for an individual Reiki session, is the practice of mindfulness. The thing is, that we do not only have to be in a state of *Gassho* in order to live a mindful lifestyle.

Living holistically and in connection with the energies of the Universe is to live in the moment. It is letting go of the past, as we cannot change that. It is not focusing on the future, as the future is not yet here, and based on what we do today, events may change for tomorrow. It is about letting go and learning to see things, and life, from an objective standpoint.

It is about letting go of judgement, and not allowing ourselves to perceive things as "good" or "bad", but accept that they are and use our tools and skills to make the best of any situation that comes our way or into our lives. It is about remembering to focus on the now, and retain our focus in the present aspects of life and gain as much as we can from one moment, before moving to the next.

Meditation helps with this. Meditation on the five principles of Reiki will truly help you to let go of those things that have no place in your life, and to open yourself to those things that do need to be there.

We have all been told, "your body is a temple". And it is. Treat it is such. It is a temple for the conduit of the powerful and healing Universal Life Force and Reiki energies. Focus on that connection, realize the power that it holds, and how it connects to you and your body. Keep yourself mindful to what it is telling you of its needs. Focus on your health. You are less beneficial for the healing of others, if you cannot first keep yourself in a state of health. This is one of the very first principles of Reiki.

With the need to keep your body in a state of health, try to monitor what goes into your body. This is not just talking about the Reiki energy. This includes your consumption intake of food. Your body needs to be strong and healthy to be the best conduit that you can.

Foods without preservatives, eating from home instead of from fast food chains, eating fresh fruits, vegetables, and meat instead of packaged and dried or pre-prepared. By eating clean, you keep your body cleaner for the energies to better channel through you and effect the greatest and highest healing possible.

In addition to the food we put in our bodies, it is also important to keep our bodies moving instead of stagnant. When we stagnate, from just sitting, even if it is in a desk chair in our office, or sitting watching television, our energy flow stagnates as well. Spend some time daily to keep your body moving, in turn, keeping the energy moving through your body. Even if it is just as simple as going for a walk, or doing some stretches while sitting in that chair... all of it moves the energy through our system and keeps it flowing for our better health.

Bringing or putting clean emotional energy into ourselves is important as well. Letting go of negative emotions, including relationships that continually bring the possibility of negative emotions or negative mental states into our lives can be crucial.

It is very hard to let go of the depth of those emotions when preparing for a Reiki session, so try to minimize the impact of these things, and these types of relationships, in your life to begin with. Try to focus on those emotions and people that bring positive energy and emotions into your life.

Allow yourself the possibility to grow beyond what you are in the now. Take stock of yourself, be mindful of those places in your life that you may feel need change, or a move from stagnation to energy. Take each one, one step at a time, and allow change to affect your life for the positive.

Take enjoyment in all that you can from life. Be respectful of yourself and others. There is always a silver lining to be found in every dark situation. Open yourself to the possibility and find it, and release that which may be holding you back from positive change and movement.

Connect with others, and with the Universal energy that connects us all. It becomes easier to live a holistic and positive lifestyle when you surround yourself with others who do the same.

Meditate daily! Whether it is on the five principles of Reiki, connecting yourself to *Gassho* and continuing to familiarize yourself with the energy of the Reiki symbols, or just simple, mindful meditation to focus on your breathing and bring yourself to a healthier state of being, be consistent in your meditation. By keeping yourself in a less stressed, more relaxed state of mind and being, you open yourself up too many possibilities and to the soundness of judgement that comes from the confidence instilled in you through your connection to the Universal energies.

By keeping your focus on your life mindful, and in the realization that everything you do effects the energy you channel through your body, by keeping with a holistic lifestyle, you are in a constant state of preparation for channeling the healing energy in the highest, best, and most effective way possible.

Reiki for Food

We started the discussion of how food can make a difference in the energy levels and cleanliness of your body in order to channel the Reiki energy. Now we're going to take that a step further. Food is much more than just nutrients and fuel added to keep our physical bodies running. Food is actually a major source of the Life Force energy that we receive from the Universe.

Food has a life force energy source all of its own. Fresher foods that help to create healthier bodies, do so because they are a stronger source of this life force energy. At one point in time, everything that we digest was alive, and all living things have their own connection to the initial source of Life Force energy that we channel when we are practicing Reiki.

Of course, the less fresh and more processed the food, the lower the levels of inherent energy still resides within, but it is still there. The problem is that while the fresher, more organic foods have high levels of energy that help to replenish our own, the more heavily processed and less natural foods, while still possessed of this energy, take longer for our bodies to digest and process, and thus can actually deplete our energy levels y trying to process them in the first place.

So, the best option, evidently, is to eat those foods that have the highest amount of Life Force energy in them. However, that still may not be enough to keep what we need in the form of energy for our bodies replenished to the levels that we actually need. Sometimes those food that we think would be high in that energy, may not have as high of energy levels as we think, for one reason or another.

Take animal products, particularly meat, for example. Animal are a very high source of Life Force energy. More so, sometimes, than humans themselves, because they live their lives without all of mental and emotional complexities that we do. Left to their own, they also eat fresher and higher sources of Life Force energy in their own foods.

Because of the preparation of meat in the way of getting it to us in the first place involves killing the animal, which changes energies into those of fear, anger, pain... it lessens, and in some cases, completely negates them as a true source of Life Force energy, if we are looking at it from a source of energy consumption, rather than as a simple state of fuel for the body.

Our own energy bodies then have to work overtime to process the negative energies into something more useful and cleaner in our systems, sometimes taking more energy from us than we are receiving in return. This may not be worth it, when viewed from this level.

All levels of contact from the initial source of the living energy to our plates effects the levels of Life Force energy contained within by the time it arrives. All of the people touching it, from the laborers gathering it, to processing it, transporting it, preparing it... even how it is cooked and who it is cooked by can have an effect on the amount of energy that our food still contains within. The emotions and mindsets of those involved, the practices and pollutants involved... it all can have its impact.

But just like us humans, there is, or was once, a store of Life Force energy available, and thus, these levels of energy can be restored and replenished. In essence, you are "blessing" your food with the Reiki energy, and transforming the energy within it for your consumption.

No, it will not make fast food healthy again to eat! (A little humor injection.) But a serious disclaimer... it also does not make food you are allergic to safe to eat again, or eliminate the possibility of food poisoning. Play as safe as you would any time you eat. What it can do, however, is to reinfuse the original Life Force energy back into the food, and help to reduce or eliminate any of the negative impact that may have affected it along the way to your plate.

If you eliminate the "in-between" people coming into contact with your food, you can simply grow your own. If you choose this option, use the Reiki energy on your plants as they grow. The energy soaked up by the plants becomes infused into the meal you create from them after.

Food preparation is another place where you can work wonders with Reiki. Microwaves can be very damaging to any energies, so you may first wish to choose to not use that as a method when you are preparing food for consumption. While you are preparing your meal, try using the *Sei Hei Ki* mental/emotional Reiki symbol over your food while in the midst of preparing it. This will help to remove negative effects previously incurred with your food. If you follow that with the use of the *Cho Ku Rei* symbol, you increase the level of energy and positive benefits that will come of it through your consumption.

If you are not the one who prepared your meal, you can always use the same Reiki energy on your food before eating, especially when dining out. If you do not wish to draw attention, or offend someone else, your drawing of the Reiki symbols can be mental, visualizing their presence in your mind. This is just as effective for infusing the symbol to your food.

If you forget to use Reiki on your food, you can always Reiki the food while it's in your stomach.

Simply place your hands on your stomach, and infuse the food within with the Reiki energy. This can also help with the digestion, especially if you feel you may have eaten a little too much!

Even if you are not attuned to Reiki and the use of the Reiki symbols and energy yet, you can still recharge and infuse your food with Life Force energy. A large part of Reiki, because of the need to let the energies do as they will for the greatest and highest good, is all about intention. Place your hands and visual the white light of the Universal Life Force infusing your food with energy and goodness, removing the negative and impure energies from it. You will find that with true intention, your food will provide you with a much higher source of Life Force energy than you have been used to!

This is only one more way of connecting to the Universe and to everything around you. It is another way of living more holistically and in tune with the Reiki and Life Force energies of the Universe. Make it a part of your lifestyle to replenish and increase your connection in every way that you can.

Healing Ourselves and Others with Reiki

Healing yourself first is the cornerstone of the Reiki initiate. You cannot affect a true heling on others until you first heal yourself. When you start healing with Reiki, you learn how to tap into the Universal Life Force energies and guide the Reiki energy through the use of the Reiki symbols. This creates beneficial changes and health for our patients, but first we must start with ourselves.

However, the manner in which we heal ourselves is very much the same in which we will use to heal others. The same focus, the same energy, the same way to call it in. The only difference is whether we direct this energy and listen for the Divine Guidance to use it for ourselves, or for someone else. In healing ourselves, we are both the vessel, or conduit, and the target for which the Reiki energy to perform its healing.

We start with *Gassho*, as described in our previous chapter on the 3 Pillars of Reiki. *Gassho* helps to bring mindfulness to our energy use, whether it is for ourselves or for others. When we feel attuned to the energy, and aware and focused on what we are doing, letting the ego fall aside and allow ourselves to be open for Divine Guidance in what we are about to do, we then move into Reiji-Ho, the calling in of the Reiki energy and allowing it to fill us.

It is here that we become the conduit for the healing Reiki energies. While the Reiki energy comes into us, we move into an even more mindful state, tuning ourselves into the energy that flows through us, allowing us to fill every aspect of our being. Here we also begin to direct it, sending it into our hands, or into our heart, wherever we choose to let the energy flow forth from us in order to perform our healing work.

It is also here where we set aside our egos, and even though directing the energy into our hands or into our hearts, we are not telling the energy what to do. By giving up ego, we are not giving up our power, or our will, we are becoming the power of Reiki itself. We become one with the energy that flows through us, so that we may open ourselves to the wisdom of the Reiki energy and do what is needed to perform the healing for the highest and best of ourselves or those we are treating.

At this point, we can begin working with the symbol of *Cho Ku Rei*, drawing the symbol on our palms to focus the energy to that point for direction when we are ready to use the Reiki energy for healing.

From here, we move into the state of *Chiryo*, the mindful waiting for guidance and direction. Because of the studies we have done to this point involving the Meridians, and the Chakras, understanding how the energy flows through our bodies, we can look inwardly when healing ourselves, or at the other individual in need of healing, and see where the energy is blocked, stagnant, depleted, or in need of repair.

This is where the pillar of *Chiryo* aids us. It is the place in our session where we examine without judgement or ego, waiting for the Divine Guidance of the Reiki energy and Universal Life Force to tell us what is wrong, to tell us what is needed. This is not something we decide for ourselves. We watch, and wait, looking for a sign as to where we are needed to direct the energy, what kind of energy is needed, and how we are going to use it for the highest and best possible healing power to take effect.

Many times, our physical ills are caused by emotional or mental issues. These can be aided by the use of the *Sei Hei Ki* symbol for transmitting the Reiki energy. You may often find that *Sei Hei Ki* is a strong first step in a healing session. When powered by the *Cho Ku Rei* energy already called into your hands, it can be of the greatest benefit.

Of course, this is just an example. It is not up to you to decide. It is up to you to be guided toward what the best way to affect the healing will be. Wait and listen. Watch. The more you work with the Reiki energy, the more you practice your mindful awareness, the better you will be at detecting these nuances of Divine Guidance that you will be given. They will be there. It may take you time to recognize and understand them, but the more you work with them, the easier it will become.

For now, you just wait. When the direction has been made clear to you, you set your intention for the healing to take place. This is also the place of *Chiryo*. This is where we allow the Reiki energy to move through us, tell us what is needed to be done, we nod in understanding, and return to our mindful place of *Gassho* to set our intention for what we are being told to do. We set our intention for what we have been told needs to be done. We set our intention for the healing with the Reiki energies to have a focused result.

Our intention for healing with Reiki energy is sort of like sending messages back and forth between us and the Reiki energy that we have received Divine Guidance, acknowledge it, and now we are repeating it in our own words to strengthen the understanding that we have received.

As long as these messages that we are receiving and sending are aligned with each other, they strengthen the focus of the energy, which is what we are trying to accomplish. In essence, we are getting on the "same page" and reinforcing what we are about to do. The Reiki energy then turns around and says... "yup... let's get this going!"

By setting your intention, you are giving the energy focus, when you send it forth to do its work. It now is in agreement with the end result, and then guides itself intuitively through the channels of your body, or those of the person you are healing, and makes the necessary adjustments here and there that may be underlying the source of what needs to ultimately be healed, even those things of which you may not be aware.

This is where some visualization may help. If you ultimately see that depression needs to be lifted, you can set your intent by visualizing what happiness looks like for yourself or the individual. If it is a physical ailment, such as a broken bone, you can visualize that bone being mended and now able to be used again. Visualization can be far more powerful than actual words, because even wordsmiths can sometimes be at a loss for those things they can visualize and yet not quite put to paper to capture the visual image they have in their minds.

This is where we can now start with the use of the Reiki symbols to actually perform the healing that needs to take place. Reiki symbols actually work to tune you in to the different frequencies of the higher energy levels needed for Reiki healing. Because of their continued, repetitive use throughout the years and generations of Reiki healers, they have become imbued with a Life Force essence of their own, that knows what to do when called into being.

Whether at this point you are called to use the *Cho Ku Rei* symbol affecting the healing or to empower other symbols to a higher level of energy, or the *Sei Hei Ki* symbol for emotional or mental healing or bringing yourself or the other person into a more relaxed and receptive state of being for the healing energies to work better, or the *Hon Sha Ze Sho Nen* for healing at a distance, or even the master symbol, *Dai Ko Myo*, the most powerful of the Reiki symbols for curing diseases, healing illnesses, or bringing forth major and wonderful changes into your life, listen to what you are guided to do, call forth the energy into the symbol by drawing or visualizing the symbol, and let the Reiki energy perform the task at hand.

Always remember to close your Reiki healing session when you feel that you are done, whether this is 5 minutes or an hour. Close it with the *Cho Ku Rei* symbol, visualizing the energy dissipating and moving harmfully into a place of readiness for use at another time. Put yourself back into a place of *Gassho*, and bring yourself mindfully back to the physical world around you, and allow the Reiki to heal what you have sent it to take care of.

Healing Animals with Reiki

Since Reiki works with the Universal Life Force energy, we have already talked about how this energy exists within all living things, including plants and animals. Humans are not the only things in this world in need of healing. Our pets and other animals can benefit from treatments of Reiki energy as well.

Besides the normal physical ailments, we all might consider, easing pain, decreasing healing time of sickness or surgery, boosting the immune system… there are other benefits to be had by our animal friends as well. Just as with humans, it can increase overall well-being, reduce stress and anxiety, and remove energy blocks. In addition, they can benefit by an increased bond between them and their owner, reducing behavioral habits, just to name a few common positive aspects of Reiki for pets.

If you are familiar enough with the Chakra system, and find that is where you are being directed to work, it might help to know that the Chakra centers in our furry friends are not quite in the same place as where they are located in ours.

The Root Chakra is located closer to the base of the tail where it meets the body. The Sacral Chakra is in about the same place, located in the abdominal area. The Solar Plexus Chakra is more on the back area, between the shoulder blades closer to where the neck meets the body. The Heart Chakra is similarly located, on the chest area, in the center near where the heart physically resides. The Throat Chakra is also similarly located, in the actual throat region. The Third Eye, or Brow Chakra is located just to the back side of the top of the head. And finally, the Crown Chakra is located more in the area where the Third Eye Chakra would be located on a human... in the brow area just above and between the eyes.

You would do a session with your pet in much the same way as you would do for yourself or someone else. There are a few differences to keep in mind. Pets are not apt to hop into a designated place and just lay there while you do a full Reiki session. Keep in mind that you may not be able to lay hand on your pet if they are not the kind to sit still for long periods.

Also, pets are very attuned to the Life Force energy. They may know better than you when they have had enough, and have no problem with just getting up and walking away from it. Learn to take this cue and let them, closing down your Reiki session as you would any other time.

If your pet is a bit more skittish, they may get a little jumpy when you start moving your hands around, drawing the Reiki energy symbols. You may be better served to visualize the symbols, to reduce your pet's nervousness with it, and allow them to be more relaxed and openly receptive to the energy you are trying to use to heal them.

Just as with healing for yourself or other humans, allow the Reiki energy and Universal Life Force to guide you to what needs to be done for the greatest healing benefit. You may find that your pet will love the energy and increased connection they get from you by working with the Reiki energies and sharing it with them!

Reiki Exercises for Beginners

The very best exercises that can help you to strengthen your connection with the Reiki energy have already been discussed, but we will put them here again for you to recall.

The 5 Principles

The first and foremost exercise for those beginning in Reiki is to practice meditation with the 5 Principles of Reiki. These are:

Kyo dake wa... Just for today...

Okolu-na... Don't get angry, or I release all anger.
Shinpai suna... Don't be grievous, or I will not worry.
Kansha shite... Express your gratitude, or I am grateful.
Goo hage me... Be diligent in your business, work hard and honestly.
Hito ni shinsetsu ni... Be kind to others.

And remember, this is step at a time, one day at a time.

Kyo dake wa... Just for today...

Gassho

The next most important exercise is to work with *Gassho*, from the 3 Pillars of Reiki, even when not preparing for a Reiki session. This is an exercise in mindfulness and connection. It is about focus. Everything about *Gassho* can be applied to regular exercise and meditation. It will increase your ability to keep in a place of mindfulness and focus, and increase your ability to connect to the Reiki energy and maintain that connection, as well as increase your ability to be receptive and recognize the Divine Guidance you receive in your sessions. Look back at the section on the 3 Pillars under *Gassho* to work with this exercise.

Breathing

Breathing is a major part of any meditative process, and will help you to find focus, bringing you to the mindful place necessary to work with the Reiki energy. Here is one way to work with your breathing and focus.

Set yourself up comfortably, whether in a sitting position, or lying down, whichever is best for you. Begin to focus on your breathing. Pay attention to its rhythm and flow, in and out, in and out. Try breathing deeper and slower, try breathing a little shallower, and faster. Take note of your control over your breath, and how the intensity of your focus helps to change its flow and direction.

Slow your breathing again, and start bringing your breath in through your nose and out through your mouth. Let your only focus be on your breathing, let any thoughts of other things go. Focus only on your breath.

Allow your breath to fill your body. Expand your awareness to your body and see if you feel any tension or stress in any location. If so, put your hands to that place, and then direct your breath there, moving it through your body. Visualize it as the Universal Life Force flowing through you, sending it to that place where it is in need of release to bring balance back into yourself.

When you feel this spot become more relaxed, start looking again through your body, letting the breath fill you. See whether there are any other spots in need of attention. If so, place your hands there, and once again direct your breath there and relax that point of your being. Charge these places with your breath, and let the tension dissipate.

Choose a third place and do the same. When you are finished, return your focus to your breathing again, in and out, in and out, slow and steady, in through the nose, out through the mouth.

When you are in a place of full relaxation, open your eyes and allow your breathing to return to normal. Stretch and ground yourself.

This practice works to start or end any of your meditation sessions, or it can also be combined with *Gassho* for the start of a Reiki session. You don't need to go through your body at the start of a Reiki session, unless there are points that are drawing your focus away from the energy session and the mindfulness of what you need to be doing. But this type of breathing focus will only serve to better your ability to stay in a place of mindfulness when you are working with the Reiki energy and seeking Divine Guidance.

Chapter 5: A Little Something More…

Holy Fire and Other Reiki Branches

We've previously made note of some of the non-traditional forms of Reiki. In some of these more recent forms, such as Holy Fire Reiki, students are not attuned by the Reiki Master or teacher. The symbols are given to the students by the Universal Life Force energy itself, in an ignition process that allows for the energy to come to the student without any interference or channel from the teacher. Each student is receiving the purest form of the symbol to be imprinted for their use.

We mention this because we have also previously commented that it is entirely possible for a student of Reiki to achieve higher levels of energy work and the healing processes without having to go through the attunement process by one of the Masters. It does still take work and dedication, but we also recommend taking a Reiki class to gain a depth of than one time to get completely through. If at any time, you need to stop the meditation and turn your mindfulness to the attention of the blockage that needs to be addressed, we urge you to do so, for yours or your client's highest and greatest benefit from the Reiki healing energies.

It is entirely possible that several sessions may be needed just to get passed one Chakra. Takes that time as needed. The Universe is telling you to slow down. After all is said and done, and you have been able to clear your Chakras in a healthy, yet gentle way, the benefits you will get from clearing those channels will be incredible and worth the time and effort that you spent. We will be going through the meditation from start to finish, but as always, listen for Divine Guidance while progressing with any use of the Reiki energy. If the time is needed for examination, take it. If there is more than one time that you have to work to get past a single Chakra, take it.

When you are finished, and your Chakras are open and receptive, you now also open yourself up to the power of the kundalini fire to rise through your energetic system and cleanse, heal, and empower you toward your best and highest healing.

Center yourself with the technique of *Gassho*, bringing yourself to a state of mindful awareness and balance for working with the Reiki energies. Focus on your breathing, in and out. Focus on your awareness of the Reiki energy of the Reiki energy being drawn around you. At any time that your mind is not focused on the meditation and starts to drift, bring yourself back to a state of *Gassho* and examine the issue, making the decision on whether to move forward, or to spend the rest of your meditation focus on what is being brought to your attention. Listen to the Divine Guidance you are being given.

Work on your breathing, slow it down, let the breath come into you more deeply. Breathe in through the nose and exhale slowly from your mouth. Let your breath become part of your mindfulness of the meditation.

understanding that you may not find through research availability alone.

Holy Fire Reiki has the basis, regardless of its name, of the Reiki understanding that it is not a religious form of healing. The "holy" in Holy Fire refers to its holistic and loving connection to the ultimate source of Universal energy. The ignition process, much like the attunement process of traditional Usui Reiki, imprints the students with direct access to this energy to be used in the healing of self and others.

Since the passing of Mrs. Takata in 1980, over 150 new branches of Reiki have emerged, each with their own essence of the connection to the Reiki energy, whether it is in how you connect, or the symbols used to connect the practitioner to the Reiki energy. Some put the count in the thousands, which are far too numerous to list here. Whichever way you choose, remember that there is no right or wrong way to practice Reiki. It is only a choice of what resonates to your soul.

Reiki and Kundalini Meditation

Earlier in the book, we discussed the Chakras, and how they work with the Reiki energy. Clearing and balancing the Chakra energy centers can be a very powerful tool in your work with Reiki, especially when powering them up through the use of *Cho Ku Rei*.

Please realize, that in cleansing and balancing the Chakras that there can be several emotional and/or mental issues that may arise that caused them to be blocked in the first place. These things will need to be addressed for the energy to flow properly again. As you work with the cleansing and balancing of each Chakra, take the time to examine the energies that are arising, so that it can be handled in a healthy and beneficial manner. Never try to force your Chakras to open, it must be done with examination and gentleness.

As our closing, we are going to be guiding you through a Chakra cleansing and balancing meditation done with the Reiki energy. Depending on the source of the blockages, this may take more

Use *Sei Hei Ki* to bring in the Reiki energy, allowing it to fill your body. Let it fill the energy channels that run through your body, and allow the energy to infuse itself into your Chakra system.

Focus the Reiki energy on the Chakra system, beginning at the Root Chakra. When you feel the Reiki energy gathered there, at your Root Chakra, move your hands down and place them over the area where the Root Chakra is located.

Visualize the red energy of the Chakra center. See the Reiki energy flowing into it. Pay attention to any guidance received from the Reiki energy that tells you whether or not it is flowing smoothly. If it's not flowing smoothly, then this is the time to drop back into *Gassho* and try to discover what is blocking the Reiki energy from moving without blockage through the Root Chakra.

If it does seem to be moving into the Chakra without blockage, then invoke the Reiki energy to empower the Chakra with the *Cho Ku Rei* symbol flowing from your hands into the Chakra. See the brightness

and intensity of the energy increase, feel the warmth that rises from the bottom of the Chakra moving upward. When ready, move to the Sacral Chakra.

Focus the Reiki energy now at the Sacral Chakra. When you feel the Reiki energy gathered there, at your Sacral Chakra, move your hands down and place them over the area where the Sacral Chakra is located.

Visualize the orange energy of the Chakra center. See the Reiki energy flowing into it. Pay attention to any guidance received from the Reiki energy that tells you whether or not it is flowing smoothly. If it's not flowing smoothly, then this is the time to drop back into *Gassho* and try to discover what is blocking the Reiki energy from moving without blockage through the Sacral Chakra.

If it does seem to be moving into the Chakra without blockage, then invoke the Reiki energy to empower the Chakra with the *Cho Ku Rei* symbol flowing from your hands into the Chakra. See the brightness

and intensity of the energy increase, feel the warmth that rises from the bottom of the Chakra moving upward. When ready, move to the Solar Plexus Chakra.

Focus the Reiki energy now at the Solar Plexus Chakra. When you feel the Reiki energy gathered there, at your Solar Plexus Chakra, move your hands down and place them over the area where the Solar Plexus Chakra is located.

Visualize the yellow energy of the Chakra center. See the Reiki energy flowing into it. Pay attention to any guidance received from the Reiki energy that tells you whether or not it is flowing smoothly. If it's not flowing smoothly, then this is the time to drop back into *Gassho* and try to discover what is blocking the Reiki energy from moving without blockage through the Solar Plexus Chakra.

If it does seem to be moving into the Chakra without blockage, then invoke the Reiki energy to empower the Chakra with the *Cho Ku Rei* symbol flowing from your hands into the Chakra. See the brightness

and intensity of the energy increase, feel the warmth that rises from the bottom of the Chakra moving upward. When ready, move to the Heart Chakra.

Focus the Reiki energy now at the Heart Chakra. When you feel the Reiki energy gathered there, at your Heart Chakra, move your hands down and place them over the area where the Heart is located.

Visualize the green energy of the Chakra center. See the Reiki energy flowing into it. Pay attention to any guidance received from the Reiki energy that tells you whether or not it is flowing smoothly. If it's not flowing smoothly, then this is the time to drop back to *Gassho* and try to discover what is blocking the energy from moving without blockage through the Heart Chakra.

seem to be moving into the Chakra without then invoke the Reiki energy to empower with the *Cho Ku Rei* symbol flowing hands into the Chakra. See the brightness of the energy increase, feel the warmth that rises from the bottom of the Chakra moving upward. When ready, move to the Throat Chakra.

Focus the Reiki energy now at the Throat Chakra. When you feel the Reiki energy gathered there, at your Throat Chakra, move your hands down and place them over the area where the Throat is located.

Visualize the blue energy of the Chakra center. See the Reiki energy flowing into it. Pay attention to any guidance received from the Reiki energy that tells you whether or not it is flowing smoothly. If it's not flowing smoothly, then this is the time to drop back into *Gassho* and try to discover what is blocking the Reiki energy from moving without blockage through the Throat Chakra.

If it does seem to be moving into the Chakra without blockage, then invoke the Reiki energy to empower the Chakra with the *Cho Ku Rei* symbol flowing from your hands into the Chakra. See the brightness and intensity of the energy increase, feel the

warmth that rises from the bottom of the Chakra moving upward. When ready, move to the Third Eye or Brow Chakra.

Focus the Reiki energy now at the Third Eye Chakra. When you feel the Reiki energy gathered there, at your Third Eye Chakra, move your hands down and place them over the area where the Third Eye is located.

Visualize the indigo energy of the Chakra center. See the Reiki energy flowing into it. Pay attention to any guidance received from the Reiki energy that tells you whether or not it is flowing smoothly. If it's not flowing smoothly, then this is the time to drop back into *Gassho* and try to discover what is blocking the Reiki energy from moving without blockage through the Third Eye Chakra.

If it does seem to be moving into the Chakra without blockage, then invoke the Reiki energy to empower the Chakra with the *Cho Ku Rei* symbol flowing from your hands into the Chakra. See the brightness and intensity of the energy increase, feel the

warmth that rises from the bottom of the Chakra moving upward. When ready, move to the Crown Chakra.

Focus the Reiki energy now at the Crown Chakra. When you feel the Reiki energy gathered there, at your Crown Chakra, move your hands down and place them over the area where the Crown is located.

Visualize the violet energy of the Chakra center. See the Reiki energy flowing into it. Pay attention to any guidance received from the Reiki energy that tells you whether or not it is flowing smoothly. If it's not flowing smoothly, then this is the time to drop back into *Gassho* and try to discover what is blocking the Reiki energy from moving without blockage through the Crown Chakra.

If it does seem to be moving into the Chakra without blockage, then invoke the Reiki energy to empower the Chakra with the Cho Ku Rei symbol flowing from your hands into the Chakra. See the brightness and intensity of the energy increase, feel the warmth that rises from the bottom of the Chakra moving upward.

When you have reached this point, and all of the Chakras are open, focus again on the warmth of the energy that you brought up through the Chakras. Reach back down to the source of that energy, coiled around the Root Chakra. This is the kundalini energy of the Chakra system.

This energy lies coiled, like a serpent, waiting to be called forth. Using the *Cho Ku Rei* symbol, bring the spiral of the *Cho Ku Rei* into 3-dimensional space by taking the spiral upward through your body. Instead of visualizing it as a flat spiral, see that spiral pass through each of the Chakras as it moves upward, drawing the power of the kundalini with it, the fire serpent of energy rising from the Root Chakra and through each of the Chakra centers, until it pours outward from your Crown.

Spend some time in this moment, enjoying the ultimate connection of the root base of your personal energy reaching out to touch that of the and intensity of the energy increase, feel the warmth that rises from the bottom of the Chakra moving upward. When ready, move to the Solar Plexus Chakra.

Focus the Reiki energy now at the Solar Plexus Chakra. When you feel the Reiki energy gathered there, at your Solar Plexus Chakra, move your hands down and place them over the area where the Solar Plexus Chakra is located.

Visualize the yellow energy of the Chakra center. See the Reiki energy flowing into it. Pay attention to any guidance received from the Reiki energy that tells you whether or not it is flowing smoothly. If it's not flowing smoothly, then this is the time to drop back into *Gassho* and try to discover what is blocking the Reiki energy from moving without blockage through the Solar Plexus Chakra.

If it does seem to be moving into the Chakra without blockage, then invoke the Reiki energy to empower the Chakra with the *Cho Ku Rei* symbol flowing from your hands into the Chakra. See the brightness

and intensity of the energy increase, feel the warmth that rises from the bottom of the Chakra moving upward. When ready, move to the Heart Chakra.

Focus the Reiki energy now at the Heart Chakra. When you feel the Reiki energy gathered there, at your Heart Chakra, move your hands down and place them over the area where the Heart is located.

Visualize the green energy of the Chakra center. See the Reiki energy flowing into it. Pay attention to any guidance received from the Reiki energy that tells you whether or not it is flowing smoothly. If it's not flowing smoothly, then this is the time to drop back into *Gassho* and try to discover what is blocking the Reiki energy from moving without blockage through the Heart Chakra.

If it does seem to be moving into the Chakra without blockage, then invoke the Reiki energy to empower the Chakra with the *Cho Ku Rei* symbol flowing from your hands into the Chakra. See the brightness and intensity of the energy increase, feel the

Divine Universal energy. Listen to what it tells you. Pay attention to the Divine Guidance being offered.

When you are ready, and you feel that your meditation has reached a conclusion, or, if for some reason, you feel any sense of being overwhelmed, don't panic. Return to your state of *Gassho*. Ground yourself and refocus your mindfulness to yourself, Pull back from the Universal energy and gentle close the channel, allowing the kundalini fire serpent to slip back down into its resting state again, knowing that you can call it forth at a later time, any time you need the power of its connection.

Close your meditation as you would with any Reiki session, by releasing the Reiki energy and giving thanks for your work with it on that day.

Conclusion

Thank you for making it through to the end of *Reiki Healing*, let's hope it was informative and able to provide you with all of the tools you need to achieve your goals whatever they may be.

The next step is to start practicing the techniques that you learned within.

Reiki is a powerful and personal tool for healing. It allows you to do things that might not otherwise be possible, by opening yourself and connecting the Divine Universe and receiving guidance and techniques that might not otherwise be known to others.

As with any modality that deals with anything, not just that of energy work, it takes time and practice. Just as with any other relationship, you need to work with it and discover how you best can work with each other. It is a dance of the Divine, a connection to a source of pure life and energy. And it can all be yours.

Finally, if you found this book useful in any way, a review on Amazon is always appreciated!